Frontiers of Radiation Therapy and Oncology

Vol. 38

Series Editors

J.L. Meyer   *San Francisco, Calif.*
W. Hinkelbein   *Berlin*

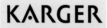

6th International Symposium on Special Aspects of Radiotherapy,
Berlin, September 5–7, 2002

....

Controversies in Gastrointestinal Tumor Therapy

Volume Editors

T. Wiegel *Berlin*
S. Höcht *Berlin*
M. Sternemann *Berlin*
H.J. Buhr *Berlin*
W. Hinkelbein *Berlin*

43 figures, 6 in color, and 10 tables, 2004

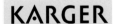
Basel · Freiburg · Paris · London · New York ·
Bangalore · Bangkok · Singapore · Tokyo · Sydney

Frontiers of Radiation Therapy and Oncology

Founded 1968 by J.M. Vaeth, San Francisco, Calif.

....

Prof. Dr. T. Wiegel

Charité – Campus Benjamin Franklin
Department of Radiology
Berlin (Germany)

Library of Congress Cataloging-in-Publication Data

International Symposium on Special Aspects of Radiotherapy (6th : 2002: Berlin, Germany)
  Controversies in gastrointestinal tumor therapy / 6th International Symposium on Special Aspects of
  Radiotherapy, Berlin, September 5–7, 2002; vol. editors, T. Wiegel ... [et al.].
    p.: cm. – (Frontiers of radiation therapy and oncology, ISSN 0071–9676 ; v. 38)
  Includes bibliographical references and index.
  ISBN 3–8055–7690–0
  1. Rectum–Cancer–Radiotherapy–Congresses.   2. Pancreas–Cancer–Radiotherapy–Congresses.
  3. Liver metastasis–Radiotherapy–Congresses.   I. Wiegel, T.   II. Title.   III. Series.
  RC280.R37I55 2002
  616.99′4330642–dc22

                                                                                    2004043473

    Bibliographic Indices. This publication is listed in bibliographic services, including Current Contents® and
Index Medicus.

© Copyright 2004 by S. Karger AG, P.O. Box, CH–4009 Basel (Switzerland)
www.karger.com
Printed in Switzerland on acid-free paper by Reinhardt Druck, Basel
ISSN 0071–9676
ISBN 3–8055–7690–0

....

Contents

Wiegel T, Höcht S, Sternemann M, Buhr HJ, Hinkelbein W (eds): Controversies in Gastrointestinal Tumor Therapy. Front Radiat Ther Oncol. Basel, Karger, 2004, vol 38, pp 1–12

....

Magnetic Resonance Imaging of Rectal Cancer: What Radiation Oncologists Need to Know

Regina G.H. Beets-Tan[b], *Roy F.A. Vliegen*[b], *Geerard L. Beets*[a]

Departments of [a]Surgery and [b]Radiology, University Hospital of Maastricht, Maastricht, The Netherlands

Rectal cancer carries a poor prognosis because of the risk of both metastases and local recurrences. Although local recurrences have a small impact on survival rates, they have a profound impact on the quality of life. A local recurrence is often debilitating because of severe pain and immobility, and prolonged and multiple hospital admissions for surgery, radiation and chemotherapy. Attention has therefore mainly been directed toward defining the best treatment strategy for the primary tumor in order to obtain optimal local control, combining radiation therapy [1–4] with optimal surgery, a total mesorectal excision (TME) [5] (fig. 1).

Because high-risk patients benefit from extensive neoadjuvant treatment [6], imaging can play an important role in the preoperative identification of these patients. High-resolution magnetic resonance imaging (MRI) has recently been reported to be a reliable tool for the preoperative identification of the circumferential resection margin at TME [7, 8], an important prognostic indicator for local recurrences. MRI has also been reported to be superior to CT for the preoperative assessment of tumor invasion in surrounding structures [9, 10]. MRI is therefore more frequently being applied as a routine investigation in the preoperative work up of patients with rectal cancer. Clinicians dealing with rectal cancer patients are nowadays confronted not only with MR images of rectal tumors but also with the complex MR images of irradiated rectal cancer. This essay provides an overview of significant MR findings in rectal cancer and illustrates some of the interpretation difficulties in MR images of irradiated rectal cancer.

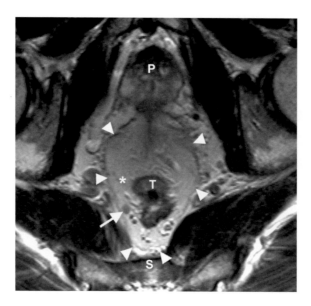

Fig. 1. Total mesorectal excision (TME). Axial T2W TSE MR image of a patient with rectal cancer clearly shows the mesorectal fascia (arrowheads) enveloping the mesorectum. The mesorectum is an anatomic compartment that comprises the rectum (T = tumor in rectum), the mesorectal fat (asterisk), blood vessels, nerves and perirectal lymph nodes (arrow). TME surgery removes the mesorectum by sharp dissection along the mesorectal fascia. P = Prostate; S = sacrum.

MR Techniques and T-Staging Accuracies

The successful introduction of MRI in imaging of pelvic diseases and the numerous reports on the high performance of MRI have over recent years caused MRI to gradually replace CT in preoperative staging of rectal cancer. Initial MR studies used the body coil. Because conventional body coil techniques showed a resolution that was still insufficient to differentiate the individual layers of the rectal wall, overall accuracies reported for body coil MRI have not been any better than those reported for CT with figures ranging from 59 to 88% [11–17].

With the introduction of endoluminal coils, image resolution improved and detailed evaluation of the layers of the rectal wall was feasible [18]. This was also reflected in the improved and more consistent accuracies for T staging ranging between 71 and 91% [19–26]. With an endorectal MRI, however, the mesorectal fascia and surrounding pelvic structures are difficult to visualize due to the sudden signal drop off at a short distance from the coil [27],

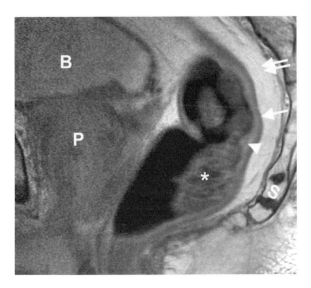

Fig. 2. MRI of T1 rectal cancer. Sagittal contrast-enhanced T1W TSE MR image showing the different rectal wall layers important for T staging. The rectal tumor (asterisk) is slightly hypo-intense to the hyper-intense submucosal layer (arrowhead) and slightly hyper-intense to the hypo-intense muscular rectal wall (arrow). There is tumor invasion in the submucosal layer but no invasion in the muscularis propria, stage T1 tumor. B = Bladder; P = prostate; S = sacrum.

so endorectal MRI is less accurate for the evaluation of advanced rectal tumors.

With the introduction of dedicated coils, phased array coils, improvement in MRI performance was expected [28–32]. The advantages of a high spatial resolution with a large field of view make phased array MRI suitable for staging of both superficial and advanced rectal tumors. This is shown in figures 2–5, which illustrate the phased array MR images of different stages of rectal cancer.

Nevertheless the first MR studies that used the multiple surface coil technique reported an overall accuracy for T staging of only 55–65% and obviously showed no benefit as compared to the body coil MRI or even to CT [33, 34]. The low performance of MRI in these studies could have been attributed to the low spatial resolution that was used with the early phased array techniques. But even when a higher spatial resolution had been applied with newer generation phased array coil MR techniques, the accuracy for T staging was not as consistent and high as anticipated with figures varying between 65 and 86% and considerable inter-observer variability [8, 32, 35, 36].

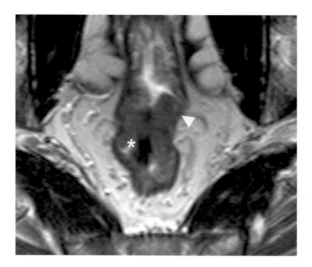

Fig. 3. MRI of T2 rectal cancer. Axial T2W TSE MR image shows a rectal tumor (asterisk), slightly hyper-intense to the muscular rectal wall (arrowhead). The tumor is limited to the rectal wall, there is no penetration into the perirectal fat, stage T2 rectal cancer.

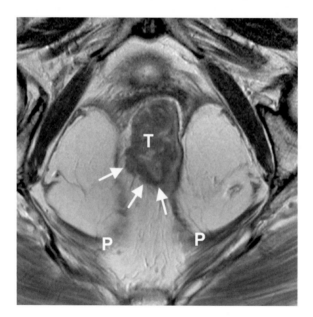

Fig. 4. MRI of T3 rectal cancer. Axial contrast-enhanced T1W TSE MR image depicting a rectal tumor (T) with tumor penetration through the rectal wall into the mesorectal fat tissue (arrows). In contrast to the tumor in figure 9, which shows a spiculated growth pattern, this tumor shows a more nodular growth pattern into the mesorectal fat, almost 100% predictive of tumor penetration through the rectal wall. P = Pelvic floor muscles.

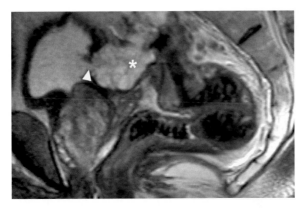

Fig. 5. MRI of T4 rectal cancer. Sagittal T2W TSE MR image of a hyper-intense rectal tumor (asterisk), invading and disrupting the dorsal bladder wall (arrowhead). This is the typical MR appearance of a mucinous adenocarcinoma.

MR Techniques and Circumferential Resection Margins

So far there have been 4 reports in literature on the MR evaluation of the mesorectal fascia and circumferential resection margins. In one study the mesorectal fascia was visualized with a high-resolution phased array MR technique, and although the authors concluded that the depth of tumor extension could be predicted with high accuracy, the more relevant distance between tumor and fascia was not studied [31]. With a postoperative MRI of 26 resected rectal tumor specimens Blomqvist et al. [37] were able to predict tumor involvement of the circumferential resection margin with high accuracy. The largest study to date on the MR evaluation of circumferential resection margins in patients with rectal cancer was published by our team in the Lancet early 2001 [8]. 76 patients underwent a preoperative phased array MRI and the images were evaluated by 2 observers. The accuracy for T staging was 83% for observer 1 but only 67% for the less experienced observer 2. For 12 T4 tumors involving the mesorectal fascia, both observers correctly predicted this in all 12 patients. In 29 patients who had a wide circumferential margin (>10 mm), observer 1 correctly predicted the margin in 28 and the less experienced observer 2 in 27 patients. For margins between 1 and 10 mm, a linear regression curve constructed for both observers showed that the crucial distance of at least 2 mm can be predicted with 97% confidence when the distance on MRI is at least 6 mm. An important finding was the high agreement of the resection margin measurements both between (intra-class correlation coefficients 0.99 and 0.91) and within the observers (intra-class correlation coefficient 0.93) in

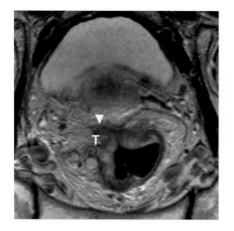

Fig. 6. MRI of rectal cancer with invasion of the mesorectal fascia. Axial T2W TSE MR image shows a rectal tumor (T) penetrating the rectal wall. There is no fat plane visible between the tumor and the thickened mesorectal fascia (arrowhead), suggesting invasion of this structure. This is important preoperative information because a wider excision than a total mesodermal excision is needed in this patient to obtain a free resection margin.

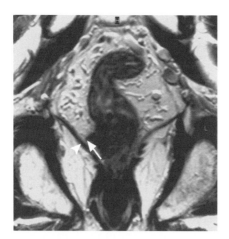

Fig. 7. MRI of rectal cancer with a close resection margin. Coronal T2W TSE MR image shows a distal rectal tumor in the right lateral wall (arrow), which has penetrated the rectal wall and extended close to the pelvic floor muscles (arrowhead). The measured distance between the tumor and mesorectal fascia was 2 mm on MRI and 3 mm at histology. MRI is very accurate in predicting the circumferential resection margin at total mesodermal excision.

contrast to the only moderate intra- and inter-observer agreement for the T-stage determination (kappa 0.53). These results were confirmed in a study by Bissett et al. [7] on the MR determination of the circumferential resection margins in 43 patients. The authors reported a 95% accuracy on the MR prediction of tumor penetration through the mesorectal resection plane.

This indicates that phased array MRI is very reliable for the prediction of the circumferential resection margin. The MR evaluation of the resection margin is more consistent and less affected by the skill of the readers than the MR evaluation of the T stage. Some of the findings of our study are illustrated in figures 6 and 7.

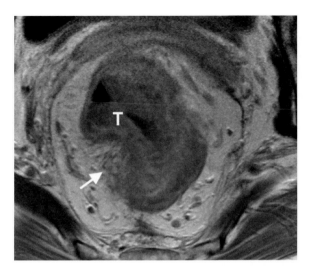

Fig. 8. MR difficulties in distinguishing between fibrosis with and without viable tumor cells. Axial contrast-enhanced T1W MR image shows a rectal tumor (T) with spiculated infiltration (arrow) in the mesorectal fat, suggesting a T3 tumor. The spiculations consist of desmoplastic reaction only, there were no tumor cells, histologically stage T2 tumor. MRI overstaged the tumor.

MRI of Rectal Cancer: A Word of Caution

Most staging failures with MRI occur in the differentiation of T2 and borderline T3 lesions with overstaging as the main cause of errors. Overstaging is often caused by desmoplastic reactions [8, 26, 38] and it is difficult to distinguish between spiculation in the perirectal fat caused by fibrosis only (stage pT2) and spiculation caused by fibrosis that contains tumor cells (stage pT3) on MRI [8]. Figures 8 and 9 illustrate this pitfall best. Both figures show similar MR pictures of 2 patients with a rectal tumor and tumoral stranding into the mesorectal fat. The patient in figure 8 had a T2 rectal cancer, while the patient in figure 9 had a T3 rectal cancer. Differentiation between T2 and T3 tumors is difficult in the case of a spiculated growth pattern. A spiculated pattern is usually caused by a desmoplastic reaction around the tumor, but MRI cannot accurately distinguish between fibrosis with or without viable tumor cells. A nodular growth pattern, as shown in figure 4, however, is more predictive of tumor penetration through the rectal wall.

Interpretation problems also occur on MRI of irradiated rectal cancer. Radiotherapy can cause tumor shrinkage, necrosis and fibrosis, as shown in figure 10 MRI can be useful to evaluate tumor response after radiotherapy, but one should be aware of some pitfalls [9]. Figures 11 and 12 illustrate some of

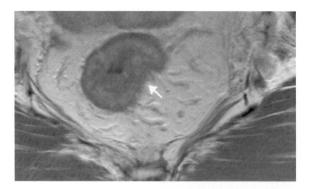

Fig. 9. MR difficulties in distinguishing between fibrosis with and without viable tumor cells. Axial contrast-enhanced T1W MR image of a rectal tumor shows a similar pattern of spiculations in the mesorectal fat as in figure 8 (arrow). However, in this patient these spiculations consisted of fibrosis with viable tumor cells, histologically stage T3 tumor. Differentiation between T2 and T3 tumors is difficult in case of a spiculated growth pattern. A spiculated pattern is usually caused by a desmoplastic reaction around the tumor, but MRI cannot accurately distinguish between fibrosis with or without viable tumor cells.

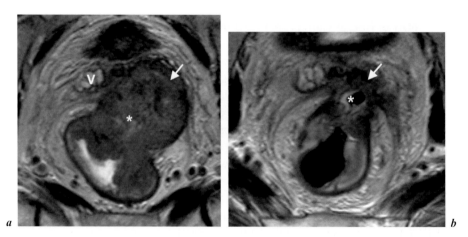

a   *b*

Fig. 10. a MRI of rectal cancer before and after radiotherapy. Axial T2W TSE MR image of rectal cancer before radiotherapy shows a bulky anterior located tumor (asterisk), which has penetrated the mesorectal fat and invaded the left seminal vesicle (arrow). V = Normal seminal vesicle. *b* Axial T2W TSE MR image of the same patient after a long course of radiation therapy. There is a reduction in tumor size and overall the tumor has become more hypo-intense, suggestive of post-radiation fibrosis (arrow). The central part of the tumor has become hyper-intense or necrotic and there is also a central crater (asterisk).

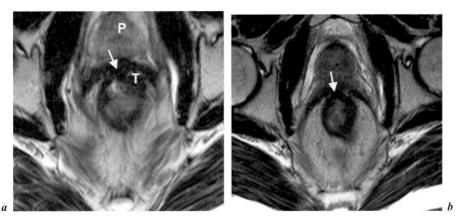

a   *b*

Fig. 11. MRI of rectal cancer before and after radiotherapy. *a* Axial T2W TSE MR image of rectal cancer before radiotherapy shows an anteriorly located tumor (T), slightly hyper-intense to the muscularis propria, invading the pelvic floor muscles (arrow). P = Prostate. *b* Axial T2W MR image of the same patient after a long course of radiotherapy shows a reduction in the tumor size (arrow) and signal intensity, suggesting post-radiation fibrosis. In the resection specimen, no viable tumor cells were detected. The residual hypo-intense mass was based on fibrosis only.

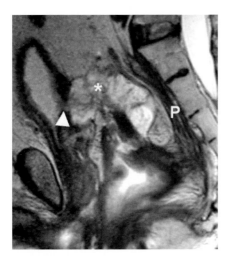

Fig. 12. MRI of rectal cancer after radiotherapy. Sagittal T2W TSE MR image shows a hyper-intense tumor (asterisk) invading the dorsal bladder wall (arrow-head), suggestive of a mucinous adenocarcinoma. The presacral fascia is thickened (P) and shows a very hypo-intense aspect after irradiation, resembling the radiation fibrosis in figure 11b. However, this presacral fascia contained viable tumor cells. MRI cannot reliably differentiate between fibrosis with or without tumor cells.

these pitfalls. A hypo-intense mass after radiotherapy generally represents fibrosis, but in some cases can contain viable tumor cells [39]. Again MRI cannot reliably distinguish between fibrosis with or without viable tumor cells.

When MRI shows these changes around the resection margin they may cause interpretation difficulties in predicting whether the resection margin will be free. In order to minimize these interpretation problems, one should make a baseline MRI before radiotherapy. Surgeons often dissect the whole area of fibrosis assuming that fibrosis on post-radiation MRI indicates a former tumor location.

Conclusion

MRI is a reliable imaging modality for the preoperative determination of the lateral tumor-free resection margin and local tumor extent in patients with rectal cancer. This allows an accurate preoperative selection by MRI of those patients with advanced tumors and a high risk of local recurrence who will benefit from more extensive (neoadjuvant) treatment. Nevertheless some difficulties can occur in reading MR images, especially of patients with irradiated rectal cancer, that prevents accurate prediction of the resection margins. Most interpretation difficulties are caused by post-radiation fibrosis. When MRI is going to be used for clinical decision making one should be aware not only of the normal MR appearances of rectal cancer but also of the pitfalls of MRI in irradiated rectal cancer. This essay has provided an overview of significant MR findings in rectal cancer and discussed some of the pitfalls in interpreting MRI of irradiated rectal cancer.

References

1   Minsky BD: Adjuvant radiation therapy for rectal cancer: Is there finally an answer? Lancet 2001;358:1285–1286.
2   Adjuvant radiotherapy for rectal cancer: A systematic overview of 8,507 patients from 22 randomised trials. Lancet 2001;358:1291–1304.
3   Swedish Rectal Cancer Trial: Improved survival with preoperative radiotherapy in resectable rectal cancer. N Engl J Med 1997;336:980–987. Published erratum: N Engl J Med 1997;336: 1539.
4   Kapiteijn E, Marijnen CA, Nagtegaal ID, Putter H, Steup WH, Wiggers T, Rutten HJ, Pahlman L, Glimelius B, van Krieken JH, Leer JW, van de Velde CJ: Preoperative radiotherapy combined with total mesorectal excision for resectable rectal cancer. N Engl J Med 2001;345:638–646.
5   Heald RJ, Ryall RD: Recurrence and survival after total mesorectal excision for rectal cancer. Lancet 1986;i:1479–1482.
6   Chen ET, Mohiuddin M, Brodovsky H, Fishbein G, Marks G: Downstaging of advanced rectal cancer following combined preoperative chemotherapy and high dose radiation. Int J Radiat Oncol Biol Phys 1994;30:169–175.
7   Bissett IP, Fernando CC, Hough DM, Cowan BR, Chau KY, Young AA, Parry BR, Hill GL: Identification of the fascia propria by magnetic resonance imaging and its relevance to preoperative assessment of rectal cancer. Dis Colon Rectum 2001;44:259–265.
8   Beets-Tan RG, Beets GL, Vliegen RF, Kessels AG, Van Boven H, De Bruine A, von Meyenfeldt MF, Baeten CG, van Engelshoven JM: Accuracy of magnetic resonance imaging in prediction of tumour-free resection margin in rectal cancer surgery. Lancet 2001;357:497–504.

9 Beets-Tan RG, Beets GL, Borstlap AC, Oei TK, Teune TM, von Meyenfeldt MF, van Engelshoven JM: Preoperative assessment of local tumor extent in advanced rectal cancer: CT or high-resolution MRI? Abdom Imaging 2000;25:533–541.

10 Blomqvist L, Holm T, Nyren S, Svanstrom R, Ulvskog Y, Iselius L: MR Imaging and computed tomography in patients with rectal tumours clinically judged as locally advanced. Clin Radiol 2002;57:211–218.

11 Butch RJ, Stark DD, Wittenberg J, Tepper JE, Saini S, Simeone JF, Mueller PR, Ferrucci JT Jr: Staging rectal cancer by MR and CT. AJR Am J Roentgenol 1986;146:1155–1560.

12 Hodgman CG, MacCarty RL, Wolff BG, May GR, Berquist TH, Sheedy PF 2nd, Beart RW Jr, Spencer RJ: Preoperative staging of rectal carcinoma by computed tomography and 0.15T magnetic resonance imaging. Preliminary report. Dis Colon Rectum 1986;29:446–450.

13 Guinet C, Buy JN, Ghossain MA, Sezeur A, Mallet A, Bigot JM, Vadrot D, Ecoiffier J: Comparison of magnetic resonance imaging and computed tomography in the preoperative staging of rectal cancer. Arch Surg 1990;125:385–388.

14 Okizuka H, Sugimura K, Ishida T: Preoperative local staging of rectal carcinoma with MR imaging and a rectal balloon. J Magn Reson Imaging 1993;3:329–335.

15 Cova M, Frezza F, Pozzi-Mucelli RS, Ukmar M, Tarjan Z, Melato M, Bucconi S, Dalla Palma L: Computed tomography and magnetic resonance in the preoperative staging of the spread of rectal cancer. A correlation with the anatomicopathological aspects (in Italian). Radiol Med (Torino) 1994;87:82–89.

16 Zerhouni EA, Rutter C, Hamilton SR, Balfe DM, Megibow AJ, Francis IR, Moss AA, Heiken JP, Tempany CM, Aisen AM, Weinreb JC, Gatsonis C, McNeil BJ: CT and MR imaging in the staging of colorectal carcinoma: Report of the Radiology Diagnostic Oncology Group II. Radiology 1996; 200:443–451.

17 Starck M, Bohe M, Fork FT, Lindstrom C, Sjoberg S: Endoluminal ultrasound and low-field magnetic resonance imaging are superior to clinical examination in the preoperative staging of rectal cancer. Eur J Surg 1995;161:841–845.

18 Vogl TJ, Pegios W, Hunerbein M, Mack MG, Schlag PM, Felix R: Use and applications of MRI techniques in the diagnosis and staging of rectal lesions. Recent Results Cancer Res 1998;146: 35–47.

19 Gualdi GF, Casciani E, Guadalaxara A, d'Orta C, Polettini E, Pappalardo G: Local staging of rectal cancer with transrectal ultrasound and endorectal magnetic resonance imaging: Comparison with histologic findings. Dis Colon Rectum 2000;43:338–345.

20 Maldjian C, Smith R, Kilger A, Schnall M, Ginsberg G, Kochman M: Endorectal surface coil MR imaging as a staging technique for rectal carcinoma: A comparison study to rectal endosonography. Abdom Imaging 2000;25:75–80.

21 Chan TW, Kressel HY, Milestone B, Tomachefski J, Schnall M, Rosato E, Daly J: Rectal carcinoma: Staging at MR imaging with endorectal surface coil. Work in progress. Radiology 1991; 181:461–467.

22 Schnall MD, Furth EE, Rosato EF, Kressel HY: Rectal tumor stage: Correlation of endorectal MR imaging and pathologic findings. Radiology 1994;190:709–714.

23 Indinnimeo M, Grasso RF, Cicchini C, Pavone P, Stazi A, Catalano C, Scipioni A, Fanelli F: Endorectal magnetic resonance imaging in the preoperative staging of rectal tumors. Int Surg 1996;81:419–422.

24 Zagoria RJ, Schlarb CA, Ott DJ, Bechtold RI, Wolfman NT, Scharling ES, Chen MY, Loggie BW: Assessment of rectal tumor infiltration utilizing endorectal MR imaging and comparison with endoscopic rectal sonography. J Surg Oncol 1997;64:312–317.

25 Pegios W, Vogl J, Mack MG, Hunerbein M, Hintze H, Balzer JO, Lobeck H, Wust P, Schlag P, Felix R: MRI diagnosis and staging of rectal carcinoma. Abdom Imaging 1996;21:211–218.

26 Vogl TJ, Pegios W, Mack MG, Hunerbein M, Hintze R, Adler A, Lobbeck H, Hammerstingl R, Wust P, Schlag P, Felix R: Accuracy of staging rectal tumors with contrast-enhanced transrectal MR imaging. AJR Am J Roentgenol 1997;168:1427–1434.

27 deSouza NM, Hall AS, Puni R, Gilderdale DJ, Young IR, Kmiot WA: High resolution magnetic resonance imaging of the anal sphincter using a dedicated endoanal coil. Comparison of magnetic resonance imaging with surgical findings. Dis Colon Rectum 1996;39:926–934.

28 Beets-Tan RG, Beets GL, van der Hoop AG, Borstlap AC, van Boven H, Rongen MJ, Baeten CG, van Engelshoven JM: High-resolution magnetic resonance imaging of the anorectal region without an endocoil. Abdom Imaging 1999;24:576–581; discussion 582–584.

29 Beets-Tan RG, Morren GL, Beets GL, Kessels AG, el Naggar K, Lemaire E, Baeten CG, van Engelshoven JM: Measurement of anal sphincter muscles: Endoanal US, endoanal MR imaging, or phased-array MR imaging? A study with healthy volunteers. Radiology 2001;220:81–89.

30 Beets-Tan RG, Beets GL, van der Hoop AG, Kessels AG, Vliegen RF, Baeten CG, van Engelshoven JM: Preoperative MR imaging of anal fistulas: Does it really help the surgeon? Radiology 2001;218:75–84.

31 Brown G, Richards CJ, Newcombe RG, Dallimore NS, Radcliffe AG, Carey DP, Bourne MW, Williams GT: Rectal carcinoma: Thin-section MR imaging for staging in 28 patients. Radiology 1999;211:215–222.

32 Blomqvist L, Machado M, Rubio C, Gabrielsson N, Granqvist S, Goldman S, Holm T: Rectal tumour staging: MR imaging using pelvic phased-array and endorectal coils vs endoscopic ultrasonography. Eur Radiol 2000;10:653–660.

33 Hadfield MB, Nicholson AA, MacDonald AW, Farouk R, Lee PW, Duthie GS, Monson JR: Preoperative staging of rectal carcinoma by magnetic resonance imaging with a pelvic phased-array coil. Br J Surg 1997;84:529–531.

34 Lange de EE, Fechner RE, Wanebo HJ: Suspected recurrent rectosigmoid carcinoma after abdominoperineal resection: MR imaging and histopathologic findings. Radiology 1989;170:323–328.

35 Blomqvist L, Holm T, Rubio C, Hindmarsh T: Rectal tumours – MR imaging with endorectal and/or phased-array coils, and histopathological staging on giant sections. A comparative study. Acta Radiol 1997;38:437–444.

36 Gagliardi G, Bayar S, Smith R, Salem RR: Preoperative staging of rectal cancer using magnetic resonance imaging with external phase-arrayed coils. Arch Surg 2002;137:447–451.

37 Blomqvist L, Rubio C, Holm T, Machado M, Hindmarsh T: Rectal adenocarcinoma: Assessment of tumour involvement of the lateral resection margin by MRI of resected specimen. Br J Radiol 1999;72:18–23.

38 Meyenberger C, Huch Boni RA, Bertschinger P, Zala GF, Klotz HP, Krestin GP: Endoscopic ultrasound and endorectal magnetic resonance imaging: A prospective, comparative study for preoperative staging and follow-up of rectal cancer. Endoscopy 1995;27:469–479.

39 Kahn H, Alexander A, Rakinic J, Nagle D, Fry R: Preoperative staging of irradiated rectal cancers using digital rectal examination, computed tomography, endorectal ultrasound, and magnetic resonance imaging does not accurately predict T0,N0 pathology. Dis Colon Rectum 1997;40:140–144.

R.G.H. Beets-Tan, MD, PhD
Department of Radiology
University Hospital of Maastricht, P. Debyelaan 25
NL–6202 AZ Maastricht (The Netherlands)
Tel. +31 43 3874910, Fax +31 43 3876909, E-Mail rbe@rdia.azm.nl

Wiegel T, Höcht S, Sternemann M, Buhr HJ, Hinkelbein W (eds): Controversies in Gastrointestinal
Tumor Therapy. Front Radiat Ther Oncol. Basel, Karger, 2004, vol 38, pp 13–23

....

Neoadjuvant Radiochemotherapy in Rectal Cancer: For Which Patients and Tumor Stages?

Claus Rödel, Rolf Sauer

Department of Radiation Therapy, University of Erlangen-Nürnberg,
Erlangen, Germany

Combined radiochemotherapy is the recommended standard postoperative therapy for patients with stage-II and III rectal cancer in the USA and Germany [1, 2]. During the last decade substantial progress has been made in treatment modalities: surgical management currently includes a broad spectrum of operative procedures ranging from radical operations like abdominoperineal resections (APRs) to innovative sphincter-preserving techniques. Specialized groups have reported excellent local control rates with total mesorectal excision (TME) alone without the addition of neoadjuvant or adjuvant treatment [3, 4]. New and improved radiation techniques using conformal radiotherapy as well as innovative chemotherapy schedules and combinations (cabecitabine, oxaliplatin, irinotecan) of chemotherapy may have the potential to further increase the therapeutic benefit of (neo)adjuvant treatment. Moreover, the basic issue of the timing of radiochemotherapy (preoperative versus postoperative) within a multimodality regimen is currently being addressed in prospective trials. This review discusses different irradiation settings in more recent and ongoing studies of perioperative radiotherapy for rectal cancer, and focuses on the issue of which patients should receive preoperative radio(chemo)therapy, and if so, how and when.

Preoperative Radiation Therapy and Radiochemotherapy – Pros and Cons

Among the potential advantages of the preoperative approach are downstaging and downsizing effects that possibly enhance curative (R0) surgery in locally advanced, e.g. T4 rectal cancer, and sphincter preservation in low-lying rectal cancer. Moreover, neoadjuvant therapy may be advantageous also in resectable rectal cancer as sterilization of the tumor cells prior to surgery may reduce the risk of tumor cell spillage during surgery. The small bowel in an inviolate abdomen will be mobile and less likely to be within a pelvic radiation portal, the irradiated volume does not require coverage of the perineum, as in the cases after APR, and there is no irradiation of the anastomotic region. Thus, preoperative irradiation may cause less acute and late toxicity and more patients will receive full-dose radiation therapy. In addition, a certain dose of irradiation seems to be more effective if given preoperatively compared with postoperatively, most probably due to the fact that oxygen tension within the tumor may be higher prior to surgical compromise of the regional blood flow. This may improve the radiosensitivity of the tumor by decreasing the more radioresistent hypoxic fraction.

A major concern regarding preoperative radiation therapy is that patients with early stage tumors or disseminated disease will often receive unnecessary treatment, necessitating improved imaging techniques that allow more accurate staging and selection of patients. Moreover, neoadjuvant treatment usually postpones definitive surgery considerably and may also be associated with increased postoperative morbidity.

Technically, there are two approaches to preoperative radiation therapy. The first is an intensive short-course radiation with large fractions, e.g. $5 \times 5\,Gy$, for 1 week followed by surgery within 1 week. The second includes 5–6 weeks of conventional fractionation (1.8–2.0 Gy), possibly combined with concurrent chemotherapy, and surgery 4–6 weeks later.

Preoperative Radiochemotherapy in T4 Rectal Cancer

Several institutions have applied preoperative radiation in conventional fractionation in the treatment of fixed (T4) rectal lesions [5–9]. The goal is to convert ('downsize') a tumor, which is clinically not amenable to curative resection at presentation, to a resectable status. Minsky et al. [10] compared preoperative radiotherapy (50.4 Gy) with or without 5-FU/high-dose folinic acid and showed that 90% of the patients with initially 'unresectable' tumors were converted to resectable lesions by preoperative combined therapy as compared with only 64% of those who received radiation therapy alone. Moreover, a complete pathologic response was found in 20% of patients receiving combined modality therapy as compared to 6% receiving radiotherapy alone, indicating an enhancement of radiation-induced 'downstaging' by concomitant 5-FU-based chemotherapy.

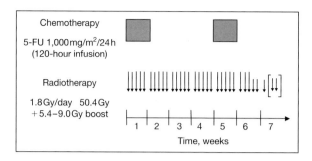

Fig. 1. Neoadjuvant radiochemotherapy regimen for locally advanced T4 rectal cancer not amenable to radical (R0) surgery at presentation, as recommended by Junginger et al. [2] and Rödel et al. [9].

Several phase-II trials of preoperative radiochemotherapy, including our own study at the University of Erlangen [9], confirmed overall and complete resectability rates of between 79 and 100% and 62 and 94%, respectively, and overall survival rates in the range of 69% at 3 years and 51% at 5 years. In a recent randomized phase-III study comparing combined radiochemotherapy with radiotherapy alone in primarily unresectable rectal cancer, Frykholm et al. [11] could demonstrate that the addition of chemotherapy to radiotherapy significantly improved local control rates, albeit no significant difference in survival was found between the groups. Thus, there is now compelling evidence that in locally advanced T4 rectal cancer conventionally fractionated radiotherapy combined with chemotherapy should be applied, although there are still few evidence-based data with regard to the optimal doses of radiation and chemotherapy as well as the type of 5-FU administration and combination with other cytotoxic agents. Figure 1 shows the Erlangen treatment regimen in T4 rectal cancer. Note that the interval between completion of radiotherapy and surgery should be at least 4 weeks to allow for tumor shrinkage.

In a subset of patients, even more aggressive attempts to achieve local tumor control, including preoperative radio-chemo-thermo-therapy [12] or intraoperative radiation-boost techniques may be indicated [13]. Moreover, as there is a substantial risk of systemic tumor cell dissemination in these locally advanced tumors, more effective chemotherapy schedules are urgently needed. A phase-I/II study at the University of Erlangen, using a combination of oxaliplatin and capecitabine together with preoperative radiotherapy in locally advanced rectal cancer (fig. 2), has already proven the feasibility of such a regimen. Preliminary data suggest a high percentage of pathologically confirmed complete remissions (21%); however, longer follow-up is necessary to draw any firm conclusion with respect to the systemic efficacy of such an intensified chemotherapy schedule [14].

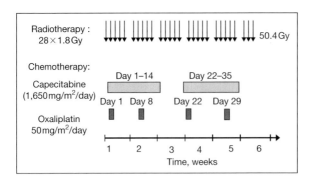

Fig. 2. Phase-I/II study of intensified neoadjuvant radiochemotherapy in T4 and low-lying tumors. Preoperative conventionally fractionated radiotherapy with intensified chemotherapy using capecitabine and oxaliplatin. Schedule of a phase-I/II study at the University of Erlangen [14].

Preoperative Radiochemotherapy in Low-Lying Tumors with Intended Sphincter Preservation

Another major goal of neoadjuvant therapy is the conversion of a low-lying tumor, i.e. a tumor located in close proximity to the dentate line, that was declared by the surgeon to require an APR, into a lesion amenable to sphincter-preserving procedures. Technically, two surgical approaches have been used after preoperative therapy: local excision and a low anterior (intersphincteric) resection with coloanal anastomosis. While the first technique should be restricted to patients with clinical stage-T1 lesions with favorable histopathologic features (G1–2, no evidence of lymph vascular invasion), the second approach has the advantage of allowing a more complete resection of the tumor and the perirectal soft tissue. It must be emphasized, however, that equivalent local control and survival rates compared to conventional APR as well as the quality of long-term rectal function is of the utmost importance in this setting.

Minsky [15] reviewed seven series [16–22] that have reported on patients with clinically resectable rectal cancer who underwent a prospective clinical assessment by their surgeons and were declared to need an APR. All applied conventional doses of radiation therapy, four used concurrent chemotherapy. A sphincter-sparing approach, mostly low anterior resection with coloanal anastomosis, was accomplished in 23–85% of patients, local control ranged from 83 to 100%, and sphincter function was declared to be 'perfect' (71%) or 'good to excellent'(85%) in two studies, respectively. However, these preliminary data need to be interpreted with caution. In a French trial of preoperative radiation in low-lying rectal cancer, the overall recurrence rate was 9%, but increased to 12% in those patients in which sphincter preservation seemed impossible at presentation, but who had an anterior resection following preoperative downsizing of their tumor [22]. Further studies are urgently needed to adequately select patients for the respective treatment alternatives.

Preoperative Radiochemotherapy in Resectable Rectal Cancer

The interest in preoperative radiochemotherapy for resectable tumors of the rectum is based not only on the success of adjuvant radiochemotherapy in the postoperative setting, but also on the many aforementioned advantages of delivering radiation treatment preoperatively. Until recently, the only randomized trial that directly compared preoperative to postoperative radiation therapy in rectal cancer has been the Uppsala trial, which was carried out between 1980 and 1985 in Sweden [23]. In the preoperative arm, patients received intensive short-course radiation (five fractions of 5.1 Gy to a total dose of 25.5 Gy in 1 week), postoperatively conventional radiation therapy (2 Gy to a total of 60 Gy with a 2-week split after 40 Gy) was applied. Preoperative radiation significantly decreased local failure rate (13 vs. 22%, p = 0.02), however, there was no significant difference in 5-year survival rates (42 vs. 38%).

Prospective randomized trials comparing the efficacy of preoperative radiochemotherapy to standard postoperative radiochemotherapy in UICC stage-II and III rectal cancer were initiated both in the United States through the Radiation Therapy Oncology Group (RTOG 94–01) and the NSABP (R-03) as well as in Germany (Protocol CAO/ARO/AIO 94). Unfortunately, both US trials suffered from a lack of accrual and have already been closed. The accrual of the German multicenter study has been going well with more than 820 patients included until September 2002. The design and treatment schedule is depicted in figure 3. Techniques of surgery are standardized and include total mesorectal excision for tumors of the lower and middle part of the rectum. In addition, stratification of all the surgeons involved has been provided for. Endpoints include local and distant control, 5-year overall and relapse-free survival, rate of curative (R0) resections and sphincter-saving procedures, toxicity of radiochemotherapy, surgical complications due to treatment mode and quality of life. First results regarding surgical morbidity and toxicity of radiochemotherapy suggest a reduced rate of gastrointestinal side effects in the neoadjuvant setting and no increase in postoperative complications following preoperative radiochemotherapy [24].

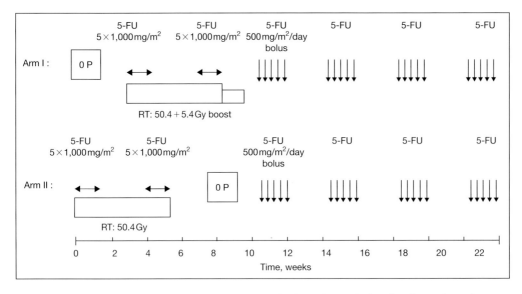

Fig. 3. Adjuvant vs. neoadjuvant radiochemotherapy in locally advanced rectal cancer. Design of the two-arm German Rectal Cancer Study (Protocol CAO/ARO/AIO 94) comparing preoperative to postoperative radiochemotherapy in locally advanced rectal cancer (UICC-stage II/III) [24].

The concurrent use of chemotherapy as part of the preoperative regimen is another important point, as it is still not clear whether data from postoperative radiochemotherapy in resectable rectal cancer can be extrapolated to the preoperative setting. The European Organization for Research and Treatment of Cancer (EORTC-study 22921) is currently conducting a four-arm trial that treats all patients with preoperative radiation in conventional fractionation and tests whether preoperative concurrent radiochemotherapy, postoperative chemotherapy, or both are superior to preoperative radiation alone [25].

Preoperative Short-Course Radiation Therapy

In an attempt to improve results in 'resectable' rectal cancer, a number of studies with various preoperative fractionation schedules, mainly intensive, short courses of radiation, were carried out in the 1970s and 1980s. The results of these trials were reviewed by Påhlman et al. [26]. In summary, while a significant decrease in local failure was shown at least in studies with higher doses, e.g. 25 Gy in five fractions, either no significant improvement in survival was observed or the benefit was restricted to subgroups.

The Swedish Rectal Cancer Trial, conducted between 1987 and 1990, was the first randomized trial to show a survival advantage for the total patient group according to an intention-to-treat analysis [27]. One thousand one hundred and sixty-eight patients with resectable rectal cancer (T1–3) were randomized to one of the two treatment arms: surgery alone or 25 Gy in five fractions followed by surgery within 1 week. The addition of preoperative radiation significantly decreased the rate of local failure from 27 to 12% (p < 0.001) and improved 5-year survival from 48 to 58% (p = 0.004). This benefit was seen in all stages. Thus, the results of this large study with a clear and simple design once again supported the oncological paradigm that survival is improved by better local control. Due to short overall treatment time, early operation, low costs and patients' convenience the concept of a 1-week preoperative radiation therapy has been adopted in many institutions in resectable rectal cancer. However, major radio- and tumor biological shortcomings have also prompted criticism.

(a) First of all, since surgery is performed only 1 week after the completion of radiation therapy, significant tumor shrinkage ('downstaging') is very unlikely and a major goal of preoperative treatment, the preservation of the sphincter, is less likely to be achieved [28]. Prolonging the interval between radiation therapy and surgery has been studied in a recent French trial in which patients with low-lying rectal cancer were randomized to undergo surgery either within the first 2 weeks after radiation therapy (39 Gy in 13 fractions) or only after 6 weeks [21]. The long interval between radiation and surgery was associated with a significantly better clinical tumor response (71.7 vs. 53.1%, p = 0.007) and pathologic downstaging (26 vs. 10.3%, p = 0.005) and sphincters were more likely to be preserved if surgery was delayed (76 vs. 68%, p = 0.27).

(b) The high single dose (5 Gy) used in the Swedish concept has been criticized for inducing more acute and late toxicity. In some patients radiotherapy-induced lumbosacral plexopathy led to an inability to walk and to persistent pain [29] – an adverse effect that is unknown after more conventional fractionation. Moreover, although postoperative mortality might not been increased after preoperative short course radiotherapy, provided more sophisticated multiple-field radiation techniques are used, acute toxicity in the Dutch TME trial included 10% neurotoxicity, 29% perineal wound complications, and 12% postoperative leaks. In the patients who developed postoperative leaks, 80% required surgery resulting in 11% mortality [30]. Conversely, the first results of the German Rectal Cancer Study (Protocol CAO/ARO/AIO 94) comparing preoperative to postoperative radiochemotherapy with conventional fractionation and with a 6-week interval to surgery suggest even a reduced rate of postoperative morbidity in the neoadjuvant arm [24]. Recent data also indicated that there is a substantial change in bowel function (median bowel frequency, incontinence for loose stools, urgency, etc.) after high-dose preoperative radiotherapy in the long-term [31], thus emphasizing the need for further optimizing radiation techniques and for identifying the risk groups for local failures to avoid substantial overtreatment.

(c) Furthermore, due to the short overall treatment time, short course, intensive radiation therapy cannot be combined with adequate doses of systemic chemotherapy. Thus, the potential of the radiosensitizing effects of concurrent chemotherapy to enhance local tumor response and to simultaneously treat occult distant metastases remains unexploited.

The most recent trial to report the results of a preoperative short course radiotherapy regimen was the Dutch CKVO 95–04 trial which randomized 1,805 patients with clinically resectable disease (T1–3) to optimized surgery with TME alone or to a regimen of 5×5 Gy applied immediately prior to TME surgery [32]. Although overall local recurrence rates were extremely low after 2 years of median follow-up in the TME-alone arm (8.2%), preoperative radiation therapy further significantly decreased local recurrences to 2.4% ($p < 0.001$). With longer follow-up, the 5-year local failure was higher with TME (12%), but was still significantly decreased to 6% with preoperative radiation. Until now, this gain in local control has not translated to an overall survival benefit (82% in both arms after 2 years) [33].

In a subgroup analysis of this study, it became evident that preoperative radiotherapy mainly reduced the risk of local recurrence in patients who had tumors with an inferior margin of ≤5 ($p = 0.05$) or 5.1–10 cm ($p < 0.001$) from the anal verge, whereas the addition of radiotherapy had no significant effect on tumors in the upper part of the rectum (10.1–15 cm, $p = 0.17$). Likewise, the benefit of preoperative radiotherapy was restricted to TNM stage-II and III tumors, an effect that was not observed for TNM stage-I and IV tumors.

This trial also once again demonstrated that no significant downstaging occurs after short-term preoperative radiotherapy, with only a modest reduction in the mean diameter of irradiated tumors compared with non-irradiated tumors (4.0–4.5 cm, $p < 0.001$) [28]. Thus, in this trial no attempt was made to select patients with low-lying tumors for a sphincter-sparing procedure and the rate of APR was equal in both randomization arms (28% for RT+TME and 27% for TME alone). Moreover, radiotherapy did not influence the number of positive resection margins, both circumferential and distal. Positive circumferential resection margins were present in 16% of patients treated with radiotherapy, compared with 19% in the TME only group ($p = 0.82$), suggesting that short-term preoperative irradiation is not able to downsize or sterilize tumors extending through the bowel wall and spreading very close to the mesorectal fascia in a way that leaves no positive margins after TME [34]. With modern MRI technology these patients at risk of positive circumferential resection margins can be identified and should, in our opinion, be selected for more intense pre-operative radiochemotherapy schedules [35].

Conclusion and Future Perspectives

Is there a standard (neo)adjuvant treatment of rectal cancer? The pros and cons have been extensively discussed in recent controversies. According to consensus conference recommendations in the USA and Germany [1, 2], post-operative radiochemotherapy remains the treatment of choice in stage-II and III resectable rectal cancer. Conversely, a consensus conference in Paris in 1994 suggested that 'the benefits observed with preoperative radiation incite to test preoperative treatment with radiotherapy and chemotherapy' [36]. Short-term preoperative radiotherapy has been widely adopted, especially in the northern parts of Europe.

New data have been collected and progress has been made both in surgery and perioperative radio(chemo)therapy. Better knowledge of distal microscopic lymphatic spread within the mesorectum has led to the use of TME for mid and low rectal cancer. With this 'optimized' surgery, local control rates have been markedly increased and local failure rates above 20% are now no longer acceptable. Technical advances in radiotherapy, including tumor and radiobiolog-ically optimized fractionation, 3-dimensional treatment planning and intensity-modulated radiation therapy will further allow application of more sophisticated treatment volumes to reduce irradiation of normal tissue and increase the thera-peutic index. Moreover, innovative ways of administration of chemotherapeutic agents, like continuous and chronomodulated infusion of 5-FU, as well as the emerging role of additional agents, e.g. capecitabine, oxaliplatin or irinotecan, need to be incorporated in multimodality regimen.

Evidently, the current monolithic approaches, established by studies more than a decade ago, to either apply the same schedule of postoperative radio-chemotherapy to all patients with stage-II/III rectal cancer or to give preopera-tive intensive short-course radiation according to the Swedish concept for all patients with resectable rectal cancer regardless of tumor stage and treatment goal (e.g. sphincter preservation), need to be questioned. The inclusion of different multimodal treatments into the surgical oncological concept, adapted to the tumor location and stage and to individual patient's risk factors is manda-tory. Clearly, future developments will aim at identifying and selecting patients for ideal treatment alternatives. Thus, clinicopathological and molecular features as well as accurate preoperative imaging and staging methods (endorectal ultrasonography, magnetic resonance imaging, PET) will play an important and integrative part in multimodality treatment of rectal cancer.

References

1 NIH Consensus Conference: Adjuvant therapy for patients with colon and rectal cancer. JAMA 1990;264:1444–1450.
2 Junginger T, Hossfeld DK, Sauer R, Hermanek P: Adjuvante Therapie bei Kolon- und Rektumkarzinom. Dt Ärztebl 1999;96:A-698–A-700.
3 MacFarlane JK, Ryall RDH, Heald RJ: Mesorectal excision for rectal cancer. Lancet 1993;341: 457–460.
4 Enker WE: Total mesorectal excision – The new golden standard of surgery for rectal cancer. Ann Med 1997;29:127–133.
5 Chan A, Wong A, Langevin J, et al: Preoperative concurrent 5-fluorouracil infusion, mitomycin C and pelvic radiation therapy in tethered and fixed rectal carcinoma. Int J Radiat Oncol Biol Phys 1993;25:791–799.
6 Minsky BD, Cohen AM, Kemeny N, et al: The efficacy of preoperative 5-fluorouracil, high-dose leucovorin, and sequential radiation therapy for unresectable rectal cancer. Cancer 1993;71: 3486–3492.
7 Marsh RD, Chu NM, Vauthey JN, et al: Preoperative treatment of patients with locally advanced unresectable rectal adenocarcinoma utilizing continuous chronobiologically shaped 5-fluorouracil infusion and radiation therapy. Cancer 1996;78:217–225.
8 Videtic GM, Fisher BJ, Perera FE, et al: Preoperative radiation with concurrent 5-fluorouracil continuous infusion for locally advanced unresectable rectal cancer. Int J Radiat Oncol Biol Phys 1998;42:319–324.
9 Rödel C, Grabenbauer GG, Schick CH, et al: Preoperative radiation with concurrent 5-fluorouracil for locally advanced T4-primary rectal cancer. Strahlenther Onkol 2000;176:161–167.
10 Minsky BD, Cohen AM, Kemeny N, Enker WE, Kelsen DP, Reichmann B, Saltz L, Sigurdson ER, Frankel J: Enhancement of radiation induced downstaging of rectal cancer by fluorouracil and high-dose leucovorin chemotherapy. J Clin Oncol 1992;10:79–84.
11 Frykholm GJ, Pahlman L, Glimelius B: Combined chemo- and radiotherapy vs. radiotherapy alone in the treatment of primary, nonresectable adenocarcinoma of the rectum. Int J Radiat Oncol Biol Phys 2001;50:427–434.
12 Rau B, Wust P, Gellermann J, et al: Phase II study on preoperative radio-chemo-thermo-therapy in locally advanced rectal cancer (in German). Strahlenther Onkol 1998;174:556–565.
13 Mannerts GH, Martijn H, Crommelin MA, et al: Feasibility and first results of multimodality treatment, combining EBRT, extensive surgery, and IORT in locally advanced primary rectal cancer. Int J radiat Oncol Biol Phys 2000;47:425–433.
14 Rödel C, Grabenbauer GG, Sauer R: Studie der Phase I/II zur Kombination von Capecitabine plus Oxaliplatin und simultaner Radiotherapie beim lokal fortgeschrittenen oder tiefsitzenden Rektumkarzinom. Strahlenther Onkol 2002;178(Sondernr 1):1.
15 Minsky BD: Cancer of the colon, rectum and anus. ASTRO-refresher course 2002, Course Nr. 211.
16 Maghfoor I, Wilkes J, Kuvshinoff B, et al: Neoadjuvant chemoradiotherapy with sphincter-sparing surgery for low lying rectal cancer (abstract). Proc Am Soc Clin Oncol 1997;16:274.
17 Wagman R, Minsky BD, Cohen AM, et al: Sphincter preservation with preoperative radiation therapy and coloanal anastomosis: Long term follow-up. Int J Radiat Oncol Biol Phys 1998;42:51–57.
18 Grann A, Minsky BD, Cohen AM: Preliminary results of preoperative 5-fluorouracil (5-FU), low dose leucovorin, and concurrent radiation therapy for resectable T3 rectal cancer. Dis Colon Rectum 1997;40:515–522.
19 Rouanet P, Fabre JM, Dubois JB: Conservative surgery for low rectal carcinoma after high-dose radiation. Ann Surg 1995;221:67–73.
20 Hyams DM, Mamounas EP, Petrelli N, et al: A clinical trial to evaluate the worth of preoperative multimodality therapy in patients with operable carcinoma of the rectum: A progress report of NSABP R-03. Dis Colon Rectum 1997;40:131–139.
21 Valentini V, Coco C, Cellini N, et al. Preoperative chemoradiation for extraperitoneal T3 rectal cancer: Acute toxicity, tumor response, and sphincter preservation. Int J Radiat Oncol Biol Phys 1998;40:1067–1072.

22 Francois Y, Nemoz CJ, Baulieux J, et al: Influence of the interval between preoperative radiation therapy and surgery on downstaging and the rate of sphincter-sparing surgery for rectal cancer: The Lyon R90–01 randomized trial. J Clin Oncol 1999;17:2396–2402.

23 Påhlman L, Glimelius B: Pre- or postoperative radiotherapy in rectal and rectosigmoid carcinoma. Ann Surg 1990;211:187–195.

24 Sauer R, Fietkau R, Wittekind C, et al: Adjuvant versus neoadjuvant radiochemotherapy for locally advanced rectal cancer: A progress report of a phase-III randomized trial. Strahlenther Onkol 2001,177:173–181.

25 Bosset JF, Pavy JJ, Bolla M, et al: Four arms phase III clinical trial for T3-T4 resectable rectal cancer comparing preoperative pelvic irradiation to preoperative irradiation combined with fluorouracil and leucovorin, with or without postoperative adjuvant chemotherapy. EORTC Radiotherapy Cooperative Group. Protocol No. 22921. Brussels, EORTC Datacenter, 1992.

26 Påhlman L: Neoadjuvant and adjuvant radio- and radio-chemotherapy of rectal carcinomas. Int J Colorectal Dis 2000;15:1–8.

27 Swedish Rectal Cancer Trial: Improved survival with preoperative radiotherapy in resectable rectal cancer. N Engl J Med 1997;336:980–987.

28 Marijnen CAM, Nagtegaal ID, Klein Kranenbarg E, et al: No downstaging after short-term preoperative radiotherapy in rectal cancer patients. J Clin Oncol 2001;19:1976–1984.

29 Frykholm-Jansson G, Sintorn K, Montelius A, et al: Acute lumbosacral plexopathy after preoperative radiotherapy in rectal carcinoma. Radiother Oncol 1996;38:121–130.

30 Marijnen CAM, Kapiteijn E, van der Velde CJH, et al: Acute side effects and complications after short-term preoperative radiotherapy combined with total mesorectal excision in primary rectal cancer: A report of a multicenter randomized trial. J Clin Oncol 2002;20:817–825.

31 Dahlberg M, Glimelius B, Graf W, et al: Preoperative irradiation affects functional results after surgery for rectal cancer. Dis Colon Rectum 1998;41:543–551.

32 Kapiteijn E, Marijnen CAM, Nagtegaal ID, et al: Preoperative radiotherapy combined with total mesorectal excision for resectable rectal cancer. N Engl J Med 2001;345:638–648.

33 Van de Velde CJH: Preoperative radiotherapy and TME-surgery for rectal cancer: Detailed analysis in relation to quality control in a randomized trial. Proc ASCO 2002;21:127a.

34 Nagtegaal ID, van Kriegen JHJM: The role of pathologists in the quality control of diagnosis and treatment of rectal cancer – An overview. Eur J Cancer 2002;38:964–972.

35 Beets-Tan RGH, Beets GL, Vliegen RFA, et al: Accuracy of magnetic resonance imaging in prediction of tumor-free resection margins in rectal cancer surgery. Lancer 2001;357:497–504.

36 Agence Nationale pour le Développement de l'Evaluation Médicale: Le choix des thérapeutiques du cancer du rectum. Conférence de Consensus, Paris, 1994.

Claus Rödel, MD
Department of Radiation Therapy
University of Erlangen-Nürnberg
Universitätsstrasse 27
DE–91054 Erlangen (Germany)
Tel. +49 9131 8533405, Fax +49 9131 8539335
E-Mail claus.roedel@strahlen.med.uni-erlangen.de

Wiegel T, Höcht S, Sternemann M, Buhr HJ, Hinkelbein W (eds): Controversies in Gastrointestinal
Tumor Therapy. Front Radiat Ther Oncol. Basel, Karger, 2004, vol 38, pp 24–27

Overview of the Role of Preoperative Radiotherapy to Increase Sphincter Preservation for Rectal Cancer

Jean-Pierre Gerard[a], *Pascale Romestaing*[b], *Olivier Chapet*[b],
Jacques Baulieux[c]

[a] Unité de Radiothérapie, Centre Antoine-Lacassagne, Nice,
[b] Service de Radiothérapie-Oncologie, CHU Lyon-Sud, Pierre Bénite, et
[c] Service de Chirurgie, Hôpital de la Croix Rousse, CHU Lyon, France

Surgery Is the Basic Treatment of Rectal Cancer

Surgery will remain the cornerstone of curative treatment of rectal cancer for many years. Important surgical improvements have been made during the past decades: reduction in surgical mortality; increase in sphincter-saving surgery with low anterior resection and colo-anal anastomosis, and a decrease in local relapse with sharp circumferential dissection of the mesorectum, so-called total mesorectal excision (TME) surgery [1–3].

High-Dose Radiotherapy Alone Is Able to Cure Selected Rectal Cancers

Since Papillon [4], it has been known that T1N0 rectal adenocarcinoma can be controlled by contact X-ray therapy delivering doses of 100 Gy or more in 3–5 fractions. For inoperable patients with T2–3 lesions staged by endorectal ultrasound, a combination of external beam radiation therapy (EBRT) delivering 50 Gy in 25 fractions over 5 weeks with contact X-ray and interstitial iridium-192 implant is able to give long-term local control of such tumors. With such an approach, the local control of uT2 and uT3 lesions is 80 and 56%, respectively, with salvage surgery possible in case of local failure. For patients <80 years of age, the 5- and 10-year survival is 75 and 60%, respectively [5].

Preoperative Radiotherapy Improves Local Control Even with TME Surgery

The Dutch colorectal trial has demonstrated clearly that at 5 years local control increased from 88 to 94% using an accelerated schedule delivering 25 Gy in 4 fractions over 5 days. So far there is no modification in overall survival and such irradiation into a large volume with a high dose per fraction increases postoperative mortality after 70 years of age and has a negative impact on sexual functions [6].

Preoperative Irradiation with Immediate Surgery Does Not Modify the Chance of Sphincter Preservation

For many years randomized trials have compared surgery alone versus preoperative radiation therapy and immediate surgery. The results show two clinical facts. First, over the past 15 years the rate of sphincter preservation has increased from 22% in the EORTC trial [7] to 45% in the Swedish trial [8], up to 65% in the Dutch trial [6]. This is the result of changes in surgical techniques and also the anatomical concepts of sphincter-saving surgery [9, 10]. Second, there is absolutely no difference in terms of sphincter preservation with the use of preoperative irradiation at a short interval (few days) before surgery because there is no time for tumor shrinkage.

Preoperative Irradiation and Delayed Surgery

The Lyon R 90.01 randomized trial has demonstrated that preoperative EBRT (39 Gy/13 F/17 days) with a long interval of 5 weeks or more before surgery was able to significantly increase the clinical and pathological tumor response. The pathological complete response on the operative specimen (sterilization + few residual cells) was 26% in the long-interval group and 10% in the short-interval group (p < 0.05). There was a trend towards more restorative surgery for low rectal cancer in the long-interval group (41 vs. 23%) [11].

Two other randomized trials comparing preoperative chemoradiation and delayed surgery versus postoperative chemoradiation are showing the same trend with an increase from 20 to 40% in sphincter-saving surgery in the preoperative group taking advantage of the tumor response [12, 13].

Wiegel T, Höcht S, Sternemann M, Buhr HJ, Hinkelbein W (eds): Controversies in Gastrointestinal Tumor Therapy. Front Radiat Ther Oncol. Basel, Karger, 2004, vol 38, pp 28–36

....

Surgery Alone: Is Total Mesorectal Excision Sufficient for Rectal Cancer?

I.R. Daniels, B.J. Moran, R.J. Heald

Pelican Cancer Foundation, Pelican Centre, North Hampshire Hospital,
Basingstoke, Hampshire, UK

Recent European multicentre trials have advocated the use of short-course radiotherapy in all cases of rectal cancer [1]. The evidence presented suggests that this modality reduces local recurrence in the presence of high-quality surgery. However, we would suggest that this approach over-treats a significant number of patients, with additional morbidity, for no survival benefit, and we would suggest that surgery alone is sufficient for selected cases of rectal cancer.

The current 'gold-standard' for the treatment of rectal cancer is the coordinated teamwork of radiologists, surgeons, oncologists and histopathologists working together within the multidisciplinary team to treat the individual patient based on the accurate staging of their rectal cancer. However, the spectrum of rectal cancer encompasses a range of disease from the early T1 or 'malignant polyp' through to the locally advanced disease involving other pelvic viscera or the lateral pelvic walls. Hence the question of surgery alone, is total mesorectal excision (TME) sufficient for rectal cancer, has to be addressed within this spectrum of disease.

For the practice of successful rectal cancer surgery and the basis for the success of the technique of TME, the crucial determinant is the relationship of the tumour to the circumferential resection margin (CRM). The status of the CRM has been shown to have a significant and major prognostic impact on the rates of local recurrence, distant metastasis and survival [2]. It may also be used as an immediate predictor of the quality of surgery and may be used for surgical audit and monitoring the value of training programmes in improving rectal cancer surgery [3]. Indeed the macroscopic evaluation of the rectal cancer specimen also allows quality of surgical excision assessment through interdisciplinary assessment [4]. Therefore if patients can be selected with a clear margin and high-quality surgery performed, perhaps the question should be redefined as: surgery alone: TME for the appropriately staged rectal cancer?

The Issue of the Circumferential Resection Margin

The prognosis of rectal cancer depends on a number of tumour factors that traditionally have been assessed by histopathological examination of the resection specimen. These include the depth of tumour invasion into and beyond the bowel wall, the number of lymph nodes involved by tumour, extra-mural venous invasion, involvement of the CRM, and the presence of ulceration of the peritoneum by tumour [5–10].

It is similarly recognised that the presence of lymph node metastases in the resected specimen worsens prognosis and this effect is most pronounced when 4 or more nodes are affected. For 1, 2–5, 6–10 and more than 10 affected nodes the 5-year survival rates were 63.6, 36.1, 21.9 and 2.1%, respectively [11]. This illustrates the importance of ensuring adequate node sampling through meticu-lous lymph node dissection [12, 13]. The practice of TME achieves this through the en-bloc resection of the embryological hind-gut 'package' containing the lymphatic drainage of the rectum.

Thus whilst individual pathological factors affect local recurrence and survival, by the en-bloc excision of the mesorectum, the only factor that the surgeon can alter is the CRM. A positive CRM must therefore represent a failure in the staging of the disease or a failure in the surgical technique.

Improving Staging of Rectal Cancer

The digital rectal examination (DRE) of a patient is one of the cornerstones of medical practice, and proctoscopy and rigid sigmoidoscopy have been the mainstay of pre-operative staging for rectal cancer since the early 20th century. However, DRE is of limited value and its correlation between observers and against other staging modalities is poor [14, 15]. The limitations of DRE are that tumours in the upper rectum cannot be clinically assessed and that DRE does not recognise the degree of extra-rectal spread or the relationship to the mesorectal fascia, although those tumours with extra-rectal spread involving other organs can be recognised accurately, i.e. fixed tumours. Thus DRE is subjective and not reproducible and cannot predict the stage of lesions high in the rectum.

The introduction of barium contrast enemas to assess the rectum and colon for evidence of obstruction improved assessment of the intraluminal component of tumours, but again had no benefit on assessing the CRM. However, with the introduction of endoluminal ultrasound (EUS), computerized tomography (CT) and magnetic resonance imaging (MRI), the local radiological assessment of rectal tumours improved. The radiological demonstration of the mesorectal fascia was first seen in 1983 using CT [16]. In an attempt to improve the image quality and resolution, endorectal MRI coils were developed. The main advantage of endorectal MRI is that it can provide exquisite detail of the anatomy of the bowel wall. However, as with EUS, high or stenosing tumours can cause insertional problems in up to 20% of cases [17, 18]. More recently in the literature, it has been suggested that high-resolution phased-array body-coil MRI staging can improve the outcome in rectal cancer by the identification of tumour invasion in relation to the mesorectal fascia [19]. To the surgeon this presents a unique opportunity, if the MRI predicts that the margin is clear then the operation must be optimal. Similarly if the resectability can be predicted from pre-operative staging then the need for pre-operative therapy could be targeted at those patients with the highest risk of the development of local recurrence [20, 21].

The disadvantage of body coil MRI is the inability to differentiate the layers of the bowel wall to allow staging for local excision. However, whilst ultrasound is accurate in the assessment of T stage, and therefore plays a role in defining patients for local resection, it is unable to demonstrate the relationship of the tumour to the mesorectal margin. Therefore, EUS assessment of circumferential margin involvement is poor. The ultrasound classification of tumour stage was proposed in 1985 [22, 23].

The presence of local lymph nodes may be identified within the mesorectum, but node involvement cannot be accurately assessed on any of the modalities. EUS is operator-dependent and has a limited field of view and similarly MRI is inaccurate based on size criteria for nodes [24, 25]. However, the significance of lymph node involvement may be reduced with the adoption of the technique of TME and the removal of all of the nodes within the mesorectal 'package'. Alternatively in some series neo-adjuvant short-course radiotherapy was given to patients prior to surgery, hence local lymph node metastases may have been over-staged and cannot be accurately predicted with MRI or EUS. However, MRI does provide a reliable measure of the extent of extra-mural invasion, which shows direct agreement with the histopathology [26]. It also offers accurate pre-operative spatial depiction of the tumour within the pelvis. With the appreciation of the degree of extra-mural spread and its relationship to the CRM, the MRI can predict areas of surgical difficulty and the surgeon can perform the operation with these images in mind. This is the result of the increased field of view compared to EUS, when using body-coil MRI. It also allows peri-tumoural fibrosis to be distinguished from tumour infiltration and it accurately depicts tumours with extensive extra-mural spread [26]. In comparison to CT, high-resolution phased array coil MRI is highly accurate and superior predicting tumour infiltration in surrounding structures in locally advanced rectal cancer [27].

It has been suggested that a phased array MRI coil accurately predicts the distance from the tumour to the mesorectal resection plane. However, in a retrospective analysis a tumour-free margin of at least 1.0 mm can be predicted with a high degree of certainty when the measured distance on the MRI is at least 5 mm, and a margin of 2 mm when the MRI distance is at least 6 mm [20]. Similarly the MRI prediction of margin was more accurate than stage [20]. However, difficulties arise when tumour deposits or nodes are encountered close to the margin. Similarly the desmoplastic response of the tumour and post-radiotherapy fibrosis cannot be reliably distinguished readily on MRI.

To address this issue the current MERCURY (Magnetic Resonance Imaging and Rectal Cancer European Equivalence) Study is prospectively addressing the relationship between the depth of tumour invasion and CRM status on MRI and the corresponding histological whole-mount sections. The results of this study will allow the development of a pre-operative staging system, based on MRI, but complemented by EUS for early lesions, and thus allow targeting of therapy.

The Surgical Technique

It is well recognised that there is a degree of inter-surgeon variability, but differences in surgeon-related variables should not be considered in isolation and differences in outcome may reflect variations in patient population and the spectrum of disease encountered [28, 29]. The operation performed may vary between surgeons, conventional vs. TME, abdominoperineal procedures (APE) vs. abdominal resection (AR), and this is based purely on personal preference, patient wishes (stoma vs. no stoma) and surgical training [30]. However, after correction for the associated known risk factors, rates of local recurrence between individual surgeons do vary from less than 5 to over 20%, thus suggesting that surgeon-related factors do influence outcome [30]. Whilst there is evidence that outcome is improved with colorectal surgical sub-speciality training, ideally surgeons with training and experience should operate on rectal cancer patients [31].

But if surgery alone is to be sufficient for rectal cancer the quality of the surgery must be optimal and there must be an assessment tool for the quality of the operation. Ideally all surgeons should be trained in the technique and continued audit performed. The first trial to accurately assess the effect of intensive surgical training in the implementation of a specific cancer surgery technique, namely TME, was performed with Swedish surgeons and reported in 2000 [32]. The basis of the teaching is the theme of 'specimen-orientated surgery', i.e. the concept that the aim of both pre-operative assessment and surgical excision is the removal by the surgeon of the optimal TME specimen, consisting of an intact mesorectal envelope with margins uninvolved by tumour [8, 33]. This hypothesis, in combination with improved pathological assessment, has been the theme of a series of workshops by the Swedish Rectal Cancer Group, the same group responsible for the Stockholm I and II Rectal Cancer Radiotherapy Trials [34, 35]. With the adoption of TME the local recurrence rate was reduced from 15% (Stockholm I Trial) to 6% (p < 0.0001) at the 2-year follow-up. Similarly cancer-related death was reduced from 15 to 9% (p < 0.002). However, there was no statistically significant difference in the incidence of distant metastases.

The effect of training also reduced the rate of APE in the study groups from 60% in the Stockholm I Trial to 27% in the TME Project [32]. The adoption of TME did not adversely affect anastomotic leak rate or 30-day mortality between the trials. The CRM positivity rate was 4% – the lowest reported incidence so far in any published series [36, 37].

Further evidence for the quality of surgery comes from the recently published Norwegian Rectal Cancer Project, initiated in 1993, and aimed at improving the outcome of patients with rectal cancer by implementing TME as the standard rectal resection technique. Over the period 1994–1997 the proportion of patients undergoing TME increased from 78 to 92%. The local recurrence rate for patients undergoing a curative resection was 6% in the TME group and 12% in the conventional surgery group. This trial also demonstrated a survival benefit. The 4-year survival rate was 73% after TME and 60% after conventional surgery [38].

Within the UK evidence for the effect of a multidisciplinary training programme for rectal cancer will be revealed later this year with the presentation of the early data from the Trent Modernisation Project, an on-going series of workshops, again with the aim of 'specimen-orientated surgery'.

To continually assess the quality of the surgical resection, a pathological assessment tool that grades the macroscopic surface of the specimen has been developed [33]. This has been validated in the current Medical Research Council CR07 trial and the CLASSIC Study (Conventional vs. Laparoscopic Surgery in Colorectal Cancer). The German Cancer Society has also been the first national body to adopt the visual assessment of the specimen within the colorectal cancer guidelines.

Targeting Neo-Adjuvant Treatments

The current European perspective is to treat all rectal cancers with neo-adjuvant therapy. These findings are based on the large Dutch and Swedish studies of neo-adjuvant short-course radiotherapy ($5 \times 5\,Gy$). The findings from these studies are indeed impressive with the reduction in local recurrence rates to <10%. However, these studies must be considered within the concept of TME.

The Swedish Rectal Cancer Group suggested that pre-operative therapy would approximately half the risk of local recurrence in any given group at risk [39]. This led to the consensus that irradiation reduced local recurrence, but the survival benefit remained unproven and neo-adjuvant radiotherapy is not without associated morbidity. The North Trent audit showed a higher than expected anastomotic leak rate (15%) and perineal wound infection rates (18%) following the introduction of pre-operative radiotherapy [40].

Meta-analyses of the currently available randomised trials were performed in 1988 and 2000 [41, 42]. The latter study concluded that, in patients with resectable rectal cancer, pre-operative radiotherapy significantly improved the overall and cancer-specific survival compared with surgery alone. However, the irradiation schedules varied greatly between trials, histological staging of patients undergoing radiotherapy was not accurate and overall complications in the immediate post-operative period were significantly increased. By excluding the Swedish data from this meta-analysis there is loss of significance for overall improvement. Indeed many of the surgeons in the Swedish trials who operated on patients with rectal cancer were not sub-specialized in colorectal surgery and performed few operations and very few were familiar with TME. Furthermore in the Swedish trials the high rate of potentially curative resections may be explained by the eligibility criteria, which excluded emergency cases and patients with pre-operative signs of distant metastases and/or locally non-resectable tumours. However, the trials showed a relative survival benefit for pre-operative radiotherapy of 21%, which gave an increase in the 5-year survival from 48 to 58% and a reduction in local recurrence from 27 to 11%. This suggests that the benefit of neo-adjuvant radiotherapy in reducing local recurrence is dependent on a high local recurrence rate for surgery alone. With local recurrence rates of less than 10%, there was, until recently, no data demonstrating a beneficial effect with the addition of radiotherapy [43]. This would mean that, in order to further reduce local recurrence, many patients would need to be treated to achieve a significant further reduction from a low baseline level [44].

The question arises as to the additive effect of TME and short-course radiotherapy. To address this issue, the Dutch Colorectal Cancer Group initiated a multi-centre randomised trial and the results were published in 2001 [44]. The conclusions were that short-course pre-operative radiotherapy reduced the risk of local recurrence in patients who had undergone a standardized TME. Local recurrence was reduced from 8.2% (TME alone) to 2.4% (TME and radiotherapy; p < 0.001) at 2 years. However, the Dutch data are only based on a 2-year follow-up at this stage and there appears to be no increase in overall survival attributable to radiotherapy. The number of surgeons and centres was high, and despite the introduction of a teaching programme for TME, 23% of patients had involved tumour margins or tumour spillage, which is of concern as the trial was for 'mobile' rectal cancers. Overall 13% of patients in the radiotherapy arm had a delay of >10 days before surgery and blood loss was significantly greater and perineal wound complication rates were higher in the radiotherapy arm, although leak rates were similar (10 vs. 11%). Of particular interest was the finding that in those patients with involved margins, short-course radiotherapy did not affect the incidence of local recurrence. The implication of these data is that radiotherapy does not help if TME does not result in a clear margin, and it may be that the effect of radiotherapy in this setting is to reduce implantation of viable cells. Thus if better quality surgery is performed, radiotherapy may be unnecessary in most cases. This again points to the greater need for an accurate method to assess the relationship of the tumour to the mesorectal margin.

Conclusion

The question asked was whether surgery alone (TME) is sufficient for all rectal cancers and the answer to this must be no. However, surgery alone is sufficient for those rectal cancers in which the CRM can be demonstrated to be clear and provided the operation is performed by a surgeon trained and audited in the technique of TME. The question thus has been altered to, 'surgery alone: TME for the appropriately staged rectal cancer?' and the answer for this must surely be yes as the key to successful surgery is the accurate selection of patients for surgery and the accurate assessment of advanced disease for neo-adjuvant therapy.

References

1   Kapiteijn E, Marijnen CAM, Nagtegaal ID, et al: Pre-operative radiotherapy combined with total mesorectal excision for resectable rectal cancer. N Engl J Med 2001;345:638–646.
2   Wibe A, Rendedal PR, Svensson E, et al: Prognostic significance of the circumferential resection margin following total mesorectal excision for rectal cancer. Br J Surg 2002;89:327–334.
3   Birbeck K, Macklin C, Tiffin N, et al: Rates of circumferential resection margin involvement vary between surgeons and predict outcomes in rectal cancer surgery. Ann Surg 2002;235:449–457.

4   Nagtegaal ID, van der Velde C, van der Worp E, Kapiteijn E, Quirke P, van Krieken JH: Macroscopic evaluation of rectal cancer resection specimen: Clinical significance of the pathologist in quality control. J Clin Oncol 2002;20:1729–1734.

5   Harrison JC, Dean PJ, El-Zeky F, Zwaag RV: From Dukes through Jass: Pathological prognostic indicators in rectal cancer. Hum Pathol 1994;25:498–505.

6   Moran M, James E, Rothenberger D, Goldberg S: Prognostic value of positive lymph nodes in rectal cancer. Dis Colon Rectum 1992;35:579–581.

7   Wolmark N, Wieand HS, Rockette HE, et al: The prognostic significance of tumor location and bowel obstruction in Dukes B and C colorectal cancer. Findings from the NSABP clinical trials. Ann Surg 1983;198:743–752.

8   Quirke P, Durdey P, Dixon MF, Williams NS: Local recurrence of rectal adenocarcinoma due to inadequate surgical resection. Histopathological study of lateral tumour spread and surgical excision. Lancet 1986;ii:996–999.

9   Hall NR, Finan PJ, al-Jaberi T, et al: Circumferential margin involvement after mesorectal excision of rectal cancer with curative intent. Predictor of survival but not local recurrence? Dis Colon Rectum 1998;41:979–983.

10   Shepherd NA, Baxter KJ, Love SB: The prognostic importance of peritoneal involvement in colonic cancer: A prospective evaluation. Gastroenterology 1997;112:1096–1102.

11   Dukes CE, Bussey HJR: The spread of rectal cancer and its effect on prognosis. Br J Surg 1958; 12:309–320.

12   Jass JR, Miller K, Northover JM: Fat clearance method versus manual dissection of lymph nodes in specimens of rectal cancer. Int J Colorectal Dis 1986;1:155–156.

13   Andreola S, Leo E, Belli F, et al: Manual dissection of adenocarcinoma of the lower third of the rectum specimens for detection of lymph node metastases smaller than 5 mm. Cancer 1996;77: 607–612.

14   Mason AY: Rectal cancer: The spectrum of selective surgery. Proc R Soc Med 1976;69: 237–244.

15   Nicholls RJ, Mason AY, Morson BC, Dixon AK, Fry IK: The clinical staging of rectal cancer. Br J Surg 1982;69:404–409.

16   Grabbe E, Lierse W, Winkler R: The perirectal fascia: Morphology and use in staging of rectal carcinoma. Radiology 1983;149:241–246.

17   Hunerbein M, Pegios W, Rau B, Vogl TJ, Felix R, Schlag PM: Prospective comparison of endorectal ultrasound, three-dimensional endorectal ultrasound, and endorectal MRI in the preoperative evaluation of rectal tumors. Preliminary results. Surg Endosc 2000;14:1005–1009.

18   Drew PJ, Farouk R, Turnbull LW, Ward SC, Hartley JE, Monson JRT: Preoperative magnetic resonance staging of rectal cancer with an endorectal coil and dynamic gadolinium enhancement. Br J Surg 1999;86:250–254.

19   Bissett IP, Fernando CC, Hough DM, et al: Identification of the fascia propria by magnetic resonance imaging and its relevance to preoperative assessment of rectal cancer. Dis Colon Rectum 2001;44:259–265.

20   Beets-Tan RGH, Beets GL, Vliegen RP, et al: Accuracy of magnetic resonance imaging in prediction of tumour-free resection margin in rectal cancer surgery. Lancet 2001;357:497–504.

21   Radcliffe A, Brown G: Will MRI provide maps of lines of excision for rectal cancer? Lancet 2001;357:495–496.

22   Hildebrandt U, Feifel G: Preoperative staging of rectal cancer by intrarectal ultrasound. Dis Colon Rectum 1985;28:42–46.

23   Hildebrandt U, Klein T, Feifel G: Endosonography of pararectal lymph nodes: In vitro and in vivo evaluation. Dis Colon Rectum 1990;33:863–868.

24   Glaser F, Schlag P, Herfarth C: Endorectal ultrasonography for the assessment of invasion of rectal tumours and lymph node involvement. Br J Surg 1990;77:883–887.

25   Katsura Y, Yamada K, Ishizawa T, Yoshinaka H, Shimazu H: Endorectal ultrasonography for the assessment of wall invasion and lymph node metastasis in rectal cancer. Dis Colon Rectum 1992;35:362–368.

26   Brown G, Richards CJ, Newcombe RG, et al: Rectal carcinoma: Thin-section MR imaging for staging in 28 patients. Radiology 1999;211:215–222.

27 Beets-Tan RG, Beets GL, Borstlap AC, et al: Preoperative assessment of local tumor extent in advanced rectal cancer: CT or high-resolution MRI? Abdom Imaging 2000;25:533–541.

28 Fielding LP, Stewart-Brown S, Blesovsky L, Kearney G: Anastomotic integrity after operations for large bowel cancer – A multicentre study. Br Med J 1980;281:411–414.

29 Phillips RK, Hittinger R, Blesovsky L, Fry JS, Fielding LP: Local recurrence following 'curative' surgery for large bowel cancer: I. The overall picture. Br J Surg 1984;71:12–16.

30 McArdle CS, Hole D: Impact of variability among surgeons on postoperative morbidity and mortality and ultimate survival. BMJ 1991;302:1501–1505.

31 Porter G, Soskolne C, Yakimets W, Newman S: Surgeon-related factors and outcome in rectal cancer. Ann Surg 1998;227:157–167.

32 Martling AL, Holm T, Ritqvist L-E, Moran BJ, Heald RJ, Cedermark B: Effect of a surgical training programme on outcome of rectal cancer in the county of Stockholm. Lancet 2000;356:93–96.

33 Quirke P, Scott N: The pathologist's role in the assessment of local recurrence in rectal carcinoma. Surg Oncol Clin North Am 1992;1:1–17.

34 Swedish Rectal Cancer Trial: Improved survival with preoperative radiotherapy in resectable rectal cancer. N Engl J Med 1997;336:980–987.

35 Swedish Rectal Cancer Trial: Local recurrence rate in a randomised multicentre trial of preoperative radiotherapy compared with operation alone in resectable rectal carcinoma. Eur J Surg 1996; 162:397–402.

36 Karanjia N, Corder AP, Bearn P, Heald RJ: Leakage from stapled low anastomosis after total mesorectal excision for carcinoma of the rectum. Br J Surg 1994;81:1224–1226.

37 Kapiteijn E, Kranenberg EK, Steup WH, et al: Total mesorectal excision with or without preoperative radiotherapy in the treatment of primary rectal cancer. Eur J Surg 1999;165:410–420.

38 Wibe A, Moller B, Norstein J, et al: A national strategic change in treatment policy for rectal cancer – Implementation of total mesorectal excision as routine treatment in Norway. A national audit. Dis Colon Rectum 2002;45:857–866.

39 Påhlman L, Glimelius B, Graffman S: Pre versus post-operative radiotherapy in rectal carcinoma: An interim report from a randomized multicentre trial. Br J Surg 1985;72:961–966.

40 Lele S, Radstone D, Eremin J, Kendal R, Hosie K: Prospective audit following the introduction of short-course pre-operative radiotherapy for rectal cancer. Br J Surg 2000;87:97–99.

41 Buyse M, Zeleniuch-Jacquotte A, Chalmers TC: Adjuvant therapy for colorectal cancer: Why we still don't know. JAMA 1988;259:3571–3578.

42 Camma C, Giunta M, Fiorica F, Pagliaro L, Craxi A, Cottone M: Preoperative radiotherapy for resectable rectal cancer: A meta-analysis. JAMA 2000;284:1008–1015.

43 Zaheer S, Pemberton JH, Farouk R, Dozois RR, Wolff BG, Ilstrup D: Surgical treatment of adenocarcinoma of the rectum. Ann Surg 1998;227:800–811.

44 Kapiteijn E, Marijnen C, Nagtegaal I, et al: Preoperative radiotherapy combined with total mesorectal excision for resectable rectal cancer. N Engl J Med 2001;345:638–646.

Prof. R.J. Heald
Pelican Cancer Foundation, Pelican Centre
North Hampshire Hospital, Aldermaston Road
Basingstoke, Hampshire RG24 9NA (UK)
Tel. +44 1256 314 848, Fax +44 1256 314 861, E-Mail R.Heald@pelicancancer.org

Wiegel T, Höcht S, Sternemann M, Buhr HJ, Hinkelbein W (eds): Controversies in Gastrointestinal
Tumor Therapy. Front Radiat Ther Oncol. Basel, Karger, 2004, vol 38, pp 37–40

·······················

Recurrent Rectal Cancer: How to Predict Resectability?

Thomas J. Vogl, Wassilios Pegios

Institute for Diagnostic and Interventional Radiology, Johann Wolfgang Goethe
University Clinic, Frankfurt am Main, Germany

Recurrent rectal cancer is a major threat to patients and a challenge to clinicians involved in the treatment of this complex disease. Currently, diagnostic and interventional radiology is involved both in the early detection of recurrent cancer and the exact verification of tumor recurrence. The imaging information obtained must be combined with surgical and oncological criteria and be verified histopathologically. Several studies have shown that recurrent rectal cancer frequently manifests as locally advanced stage pT4 in 74% and pT3 in 26%, and 54% of the patients also develop synchronous metastases. In their study of 32 patients Böhm et al. [1] proved that successful resection was only possible in 56% of the cases, or 66% if resection was extended to adjacent organs. The 4-year survival proved to be 44% in the curative group and 19% in the residual disease group. The largest study was published by Shoup et al. [2] with 634 resected patients. Resection with negative microscopic margins in the absence of vascular invasion resulted in a mean disease-free survival of 31.2 months. The group in which resection was carried out with grossly positive microscopic margins had a mean disease-free survival of 7.9 months. The authors conclude that complete resection and the absence of vascular invasion are indicators of local control and improved survival.

For the radiologist the clinical questions of recurrent rectal cancers are first of all tumor involvement with the documentation of findings such as luminal and extraluminal extension. The second most frequent question is the pattern of lymph node involvement, such as locoregional involvement, iliac-internal lymph nodes and para-aortal lymph nodes. Additional findings, such as pulmonary metastases, liver metastases or, in rare cases, musculoskeletal metastases, must also be evaluated. The detection of recurrent rectal cancer is based on clinical follow-up with tumor markers, the use of ultrasound, endosonography, rectoscopy and colonoscopy. Radiological studies which are also used for the detection of recurrent rectal cancers are the up-dated multi-slice computed tomography (CT) scanning, endorectal magnetic resonance imaging (MRI) and 2-[^{18}F]-fluoro-2-D-glucose positron electron tomography (^{18}F-FDG-PET). Three-dimensional endoluminal ultrasound is a hands-on tool for the examiner and allows exact imaging of the local tumor infiltration. However, the problem of interpretation and documentation of this technique still remains. Second, stenosing tumors do not allow complete evaluation using an endorectal ultrasound. Further problems are lymph node staging and proximal tumors. Using multi-slice CT, the diagnostic information on both the topographical data and soft tissue resolution was significantly improved. The new CT technology using 16-row CT equipment allows acquisition of excellent data sets with multi-planar reformatted images in sagittal and coronal orientation. Using virtual endoscopy, secondary lesions within the bowel might be identified in the sigmoid colon. This is based on a virtual 3-dimensional double-contrast technique. The limitations of CT are based on the limited differentiation of the wall layers. Additionally, partial volume effects lead to overstaging, especially T2 versus T3 and T3 versus T4, as well as limited information on the tumor involvement of lymph nodes.

Local recurrence of rectal cancer meets the following criteria in CT: an enlargement of a presacral mass with an inhomogeneous appearance; additionally, asymmetric outlines and relevant contrast uptake indicate possible tumor recurrence. Peritumoral interstitial radiation as well as locally enlarged lymph nodes are further characteristic signs of recurrent rectal cancer. The diagnostic accuracy is high if CT demonstrates infiltration of surrounding tissues. Data on the use of ^{18}F-FDG-PET have been published considering both the benefits and limitations [3]. While PET provides a high sensitivity there are still problems in patients suffering from diabetes with local inflammation. The advantage of PET is the fact that whole body scan gives additional information on the lymph nodes involved in lung metastases. However, PET also shows some limitations, such as long scan times, spatial resolution, which is higher than 10 mm, and the availability of the method.

MRI is a promising method. The diagnostic results are based on the understanding of the diagnostic test and the optimal examination strategy. Currently different acquisition techniques are available. The standard technique is the evaluation of the rectum and adjacent organs using a phased array coil in MRI. Additional information is provided using endorectal coil T1- and T2-weighted sequences, both plain and contrast-enhanced as well as fat-saturated. In their studies Dicle et al. [4] reported a sensitivity of 83% for contrast-enhanced MRI with the dynamic technique especially for the differentiation of recurrent cancer versus scarring. 'One-shot shopping' MRI additionally allows evaluation of the rectum and perirectal tumor lesions as well as adjacent organs like the bladder, vessels, lymph nodes, liver and basal lung. Newer technologies in CT and MRI are also helpful for histopathological verification of recurrent rectal cancer. Here two possibilities are currently available: first, CT-guided biopsy, which is most frequently performed allowing the demonstration of the lesion and the needle track. Open MR techniques have further advanced the possibilities of performing histopathological evaluation in patients with suspected recurrent cancer. Open MR allows orientation with external landmarks, free choice of slice orientation and needle tracking in predefined images. In addition, with the use of open MRI local palliative therapeutic treatments are possible with thermal ablations (laser-induced thermotherapy or radiofrequency). The current study by Pegios et al. [5] evaluating rectal cancer with endorectal MRI versus endorectal ultrasound revealed exact staging for the endorectal ultrasound of 63.3% versus endorectal MRI of 86.6%. Overstaging was detected in 23% of the cases for ultrasound and in 8% for endorectal MRI, and understaging was seen in 7% of the cases for ultrasound and in 5.6% for endorectal MRI [6].

In summary, the diagnosis of recurrent rectal cancer must first be performed by evaluating the area of anastomosis. These techniques are based on cross-sectional imaging techniques and endoluminal examination techniques like rectoscopy performed with biopsy, or submucosal endosonography. However, current problems are still the evaluation and differentiation of scarring edema versus recurrence [7–15]. Endorectal MRI as well as multi-slice CT are additionally helpful diagnostic tools in providing as much pre-therapeutic information as possible. In the majority the detection of extraluminal pelvic occurrence is based on the use of cross-sectional imaging techniques like CT or MRI, additionally supported by CT or MR-guided biopsy maneuvers.

References

1   Böhm B, Helfritzsch H, Thiele M, Altendorf-Hofmann A, Scheele J: Therapy results of locoregional recurrences in rectal cancer (in German). Zentralbl Chir 2001;126:596–601.
2   Shoup M, Guillem JG, Alektiar KM, Liau K, Paty PB, Cohen AM: Predictors of survival in recurrent rectal cancer after resection and intraoperative radiotherapy. Dis Colon Rectum 2002; 45:585–592.
3   Franke J, Rosenzweig S, Reinartz P, Hoer J, Kasperk R, Schumpelick V: Value of positron emission tomography (^{18}F-FDG-PET) in the diagnosis of recurrent rectal cancer (in German). Chirurg 2000;71:80–85.
4   Dicle O, Obuz F, Cakmakci H: Differentiation of recurrent rectal cancer and scarring with dynamic MR imaging. Br J Radiol 1999;72:1155–1159.
5   Pegios W, Hunerbein M, Schroder R, Wust P, Schlag P, Felix R, Vogl TJ: Comparison between endorectal MRI (EMRTI) and endorectal sonography (ES) after surgery or therapy for rectal

tumors to exclude recurrent or residual tumor (in German). Röfo Fortschr Geb Röntgenstr Neuen Bildgeb Verfahr 2002;174:731–737.

6   Baulieu F, Bourlier P, Scotto B, Mor C, Eder V, Picon L, De Calan L, Dorval E, Pottier JM, Baulieu JL: The value of immunoscintigraphy in the detection of recurrent colorectal cancer. Nucl Med Commun 2001;22:1295–1304.

7   Yuan HY, Li Y, Yang GL, Bei DJ, Wang K: Study on the causes of local recurrence of rectal cancer after curative resection: Analysis of 213 cases. World J Gastroenterol 1998;4:527–529.

8   Wiig JN, Poulsen JP, Larsen S, Braendengen M, Waehre H, Giercksky KE: Total pelvic exenteration with preoperative irradiation for advanced primary and recurrent rectal cancer. Eur J Surg 2002;168:42–48.

9   Bussieres E, Gilly FN, Rouanet P, Mahe MA, Roussel A, Delannes M, Gerard JP, Dubois JB, Richaud P: Recurrences of rectal cancers: Results of a multimodal approach with intraoperative radiation therapy. French Group of IORT. Intraoperative Radiation Therapy. Int J Radiat Oncol Biol Phys 1996;34:49–56.

10 Friel CM, Cromwell JW, Marra C, Madoff RD, Rothenberger DA, Garcia-Aguilar J: Salvage radical surgery after failed local excision for early rectal cancer. Dis Colon Rectum 2002;45: 875–879.

11 Beets-Tan RG, Beets GL, Borstlap AC, Oei TK, Teune TM, von Meyenfeldt MF, van Engelshoven JM: Preoperative assessment of local tumor extent in advanced rectal cancer: CT or high-resolution MRI? Abdom Imaging 2000;25:533–541.

12 Hunerbein M, Totkas S, Moesta KT, Ulmer C, Handke T, Schlag PM: The role of transrectal ultrasound-guided biopsy in the postoperative follow-up of patients with rectal cancer. Surgery 2001;129:164–169.

13 Ohhigashi S, Nishio T, Watanabe F, Matsusako M: Experience with radiofrequency ablation in the treatment of pelvic recurrence in rectal cancer: Report of two cases. Dis Colon Rectum 2001;44: 741–745.

14 Roth AD, Berney CR, Rohner S, Allal AS, Morel P, Marti MC, Aapro MS, Alberto P: Intra-arterial chemotherapy in locally advanced or recurrent carcinomas of the penis and anal canal: An active treatment modality with curative potential. Br J Cancer 2000;83:1637–1642.

15 Beets-Tan RG, Morren GL, Beets GL, Kessels AGH, el Naggar, K, Lemaire E, Baetem CGMI, van Engelshoven JMA: Measurements of anal sphincter muscles: Endoanal US, endoanal MR imaging, or phased-array MR imaging? A study with healthy volunteers. Radiology 2001;220: 81–89.

Prof. Dr. Thomas J. Vogl
Institut für Diagnostische und Interventionelle Radiologie
Klinikum der Johann-Wolfgang-Goethe-Universität
Theodor-Stern-Kai 7
DE–60590 Frankfurt am Main (Germany)
Tel. +49 69 6301 7278, Fax +49 69 6301 7258, E-Mail T.Vogl@em.uni-frankfurt.de

Wiegel T, Höcht S, Sternemann M, Buhr HJ, Hinkelbein W (eds): Controversies in Gastrointestinal
Tumor Therapy. Front Radiat Ther Oncol. Basel, Karger, 2004, vol 38, pp 41–51

....

A Multicenter Analysis of 123 Patients with Recurrent Rectal Cancer within the Pelvis

*S. Höcht[a], R. Hammad[a], H. Thiel[b], T. Wiegel[a], A. Siegmann[a],
J. Willner[c], P. Wust[d], T. Herrmann[e], M. Eble[f], D. Carstens[g],
M. Flentje[c], P. Neumann[h], W. Hinkelbein[a]*

Clinics for Radiation Oncology and Radiotherapy of: [a]Charité, Campus Benjamin
Franklin, Berlin; [b]Klinikum Bamberg; [c]Universitätsklinikum Würzburg;
[d]Universitätsklinikum Charité, Campus Virchow-Klinikum, Berlin;
[e]Universitätsklinikum TU Dresden; [f]Universitätsklinikum RWTH Aachen;
[g]Allgemeines Krankenhaus St. Georg, Hamburg, and [h]Institut für medizinische
Informatik, Biometrie und Epidemiologie, Universitätsklinikum Benjamin
Franklin, FU Berlin, Deutschland

Radiotherapy as adjuvant treatment after curative resection or given in a
neoadjuvant setting prior to the operative procedure plays a well-recognized
role in reducing rates of locoregional tumor recurrence and to some extent
improves rates of cancer-related mortality [1, 2]. Based on a clear survival benefit, postoperative radiochemotherapy in the early 1990s emerged as a standard
procedure for stage-II and III rectal cancer. A positive impact on distant metastases as well as on local control has been demonstrated [3–6]. At the time these
studies started patient accrual, rates of pelvic tumor recurrences were high and
often exceeded 20% [7]. Surgeons and pathologists searched for the anatomical
and technical basis of tumor recurrence rates parallel to the evaluation of the
benefit of adjuvant therapies, and these investigations also led to considerable
improvements in therapy [8–11].

As changes in operative therapy may not only influence rates of tumor
recurrence in the pelvis, but also the pattern of recurrence itself, and recommendations for radiation ports in adjuvant therapy are largely based on rather
outdated studies, a multicenter study was initiated to evaluate pelvic sites

of recurrence in patients treated within the last few years on a large scale [12, 13].

Material and Methods

The study was conducted between April 1998 and December 2001. 123 patients with sufficient data for analysis could be evaluated. CT image-based report forms and extensive questionnaires were evaluated with a self-developed 3-dimensionally structured CT-based data file system. Entry to the 3D data base of the complete dataset was checked by an independent experienced radiation oncologist. Criteria for patient accrual of this study were as follows. The diagnosis of recurrent rectal cancer had to be established by either one of the following major criteria: (1) histologic confirmation; (2) positive PET scan, and (3) clear bone destruction, or at least 3 of the following minor criteria: (1) invasion of adjacent organs; (2) progressive soft tissue mass on repeated CT/MRI scans; (3) typical appearance in endoscopic US, CT, MRI, and (4) consecutive rise in tumor markers.

As it may be impossible to distinguish malignant from inflammatory soft tissue masses, all patients with clinical or serological signs of inflammation or abscess formation were excluded.

For graphical analysis of the recurrence patterns and visualization of results, films were rendered from the 3D data base. Extensive quality-assurance tests were done to ascertain the exact and anatomically correct representations of sites of recurrent tumor within the pelvis. Statistical analysis of differences in recurrence patterns was facilitated by comparison on a slice-by-slice basis, thus reducing the amount of data to be handled. Tests performed were the Pearson χ^2 test with continuity correction, likelihood ratio, Fisher's exact test and linear by linear association.

Results

The initial T stage was T_1 in 2%, T_2 in 24%, T_3 in 60%, T_4 in 13%, and unknown in 1%. In 54% of the patients the lymph nodes were initially without metastases (N_0), whereas N_1 and N_2 disease (according to TNM-5) was diagnosed in 23% each. The initial surgical procedure was an abdominoperineal resection (APR) in 41%, low anterior resection (LAR) in 36% and others, namely variants of LAR, in 23% (table 1). The median age at diagnosis of recurrent rectal cancer was 61 years with a range of 32–83 years. The male:female ratio was 65:35%.

The mean time to recurrence was in the range of 22 months for T_4 or N_2 situations and 32–33 months in T_2 and/or N_0. Recurrences were solitary in 76%, at multiple sites in 5%, and in 19% this could not be defined. Clear lymph node involvement was diagnosed in 20%, in 45% lymph node involvement was absent, and in 35% it was impossible to state whether the recurrence involved lymph nodes. Invasion of the adjacent organs was quite common (table 2),

Table 1. Initial patient characteristics

	%
T stage	
T_1	2
T_2	24
T_3	60
T_4	13
Unknown	1
Nodal involvement	
N_0	54
N_1	23
N_2	23
Metastases	
M_0	89
M_1	7
Unknown	4
Grading	
G_1	2
G_2	64
G_3	28
Not stated	6
Initial surgery	
APR	41
LAR	36
Others[1]	23
With TME	9
Without TME	21
Unknown	69
Adjuvant therapy	
Chemotherapy	64
Radiotherapy[2]	17

APR = Abdominoperineal resection; LAR = low anterior resection; TME = total mesorectal excision.

[1]Namely variants of LAR.

[2]In 81% recurrent tumors within previously irradiated volume.

synchronous metastasis was diagnosed in 38%, and the liver and lungs were most often involved (table 3). Involvement of the lungs was more common in tumors treated with APR than LAR with 20 vs. 11%, whereas the opposite was true for liver metastases (12 vs. 18%).

Table 2. Infiltration/invasion of adjacent structures in recurrent disease	%
Uterus and vagina	23
Prostate and seminal vesicles	26
Bladder and urethra	11
Sacral and coccygeal bones	29

Table 3. Synchronous metastases at diagnosis of tumor recurrence	%
Overall	38
Liver	17
Lungs	15
Lymph nodes	
Para-aortic	5
Groin	5
Peritoneal cavity and abdominal wall	5
Bone	3
Brain	2

Graphic evaluation of the pelvic sites of recurrence in the 3D-computer model at first displayed recurrent tumor nearly anywhere within the pelvis, but the volume involved shrunk considerably by excluding all sites involved just once. Excluding all areas involved in less than 5% led to a further reduction of this volume (fig. 1–3). Recurrence patterns were then analyzed in subgroups of patients who had been previously treated by APR and LAR. To limit differences mainly caused by chance, sites involved in less than 10% were excluded for display purposes, as the subgroups were considerably smaller than the complete data set (fig. 4, 5). While there was no difference in the top CT slices of the pelvis, there was a statistically significant difference in the 3 lowest pelvic CT slices with results of all of the above-mentioned tests being <0.025 (fig. 6).

Discussion

Tumor recurrences of rectal cancer within the pelvis often cause pain and disabilities like fistula formation, severe neurologic deficits, compromised pelvic

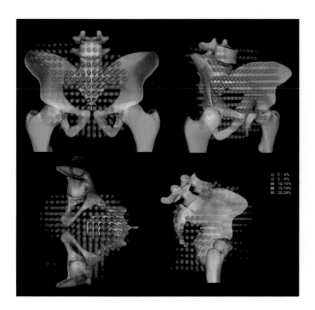

Fig. 1. Sites of recurrence in all 123 patients.

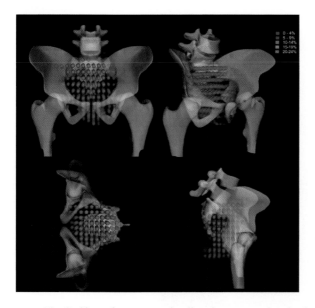

Fig. 2. Sites of recurrence in all patients: areas involved only once excluded.

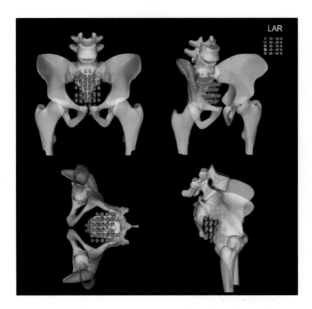

Fig. 3. Sites of recurrence in all patients: areas involved in less than 5% excluded.

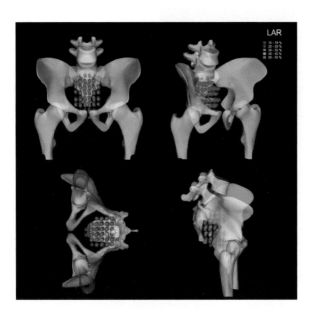

Fig. 4. Sites of recurrence after low anterior resection: areas involved in less than 10% excluded.

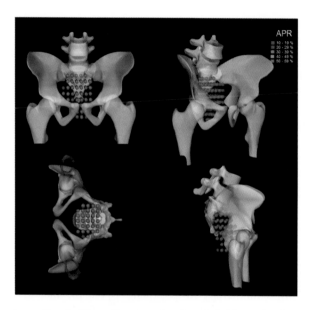

Fig. 5. Sites of recurrence after abdominoperineal resection: areas involved in less than 10% excluded.

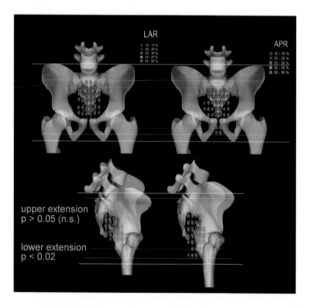

Fig. 6. Differences in extension of tumor recurrences after LAR vs. APR.

stability, bowel obstruction, etc., and have dramatic impacts on the quality of life of the afflicted patients. Once the tumor has recurred, chances of cure are small even when extensive resections and multimodality treatment strategies are applied, and only patients with small recurrent tumors at the site of the anastomosis seem to fare better [14–17].

The anatomical and technical basis of tumor recurrences within the pelvis has been extensively studied over the past 20 years and, as a result of these attempts, improvements in operative therapy have been implemented [8–11]. In large multicenter randomized studies published in the last years, 5-year locoregional recurrence rates decreased to a range of 6–18% with or without adjuvant or neoadjuvant radiotherapy [18–21].

Rates of pelvic recurrence in reality may be somewhat higher than estimated by these reports. Some studies report only first sites of failure, and pelvic relapse in the later course of disease is not always evaluated properly in patients without local symptomatic disease under palliative chemotherapy for distant metastases. Therefore, there is no clear evidence of a survival benefit attributable to the addition of radiotherapy to treatment. Given the fact that radiotherapy itself can cause even severe and in some instances fatal complications, especially in elderly patients, there is an obvious need to redefine its role [1, 22].

Therefore reducing the side effects of radiotherapy is a very important topic, and modern three-dimensional treatment planning systems and multiple field techniques undoubtedly have an enormous impact on reaching that goal [23]. Because many studies have demonstrated that the volume irradiated is a very critical factor influencing rates of acute as well as late side effects, there is no doubt that reducing the volume treated to an essential minimum is of major concern [24–26].

Modifications in operative therapy may not only influence rates but also the pelvic pattern of recurrence itself. Recommendations for radiation ports in adjuvant therapy should hence be based on the recurrence patterns of patients treated recently, but many of the studies reporting on pelvic recurrence patterns have some limitations; they are either outdated or do not give exact anatomic information on the location of recurrent tumors within the pelvis, or they just simply cover a very large time span within which changes in therapy will very likely have happened, thus compromising the ability to make their results a basis for recommendations in planning target volumes in adjuvant radiotherapy [12, 13, 15, 27–32].

The data presented in this study were collected over a short period of time and therefore represent an actual standard of care in operative therapy and, to the best of our knowledge, this is one of the largest studies on that topic giving detailed information with respect to anatomical landmarks suitable for radiotherapy treatment planning [33]. The multicenter basis of the data evaluated makes it unlikely that our results are influenced by regional specialities or the individual preferences of one surgeon or team of surgeons or simply referral practice. The shortcomings of our study are that computed tomograms were mainly used to evaluate disease extension in the pelvis (CT in 94% and MRI in 32%) and tumor spread may therefore be underestimated. Only a minority of patients (12%) had laparotomy or laparoscopy for restaging and disease evaluation. Only 17% of the patients evaluated had previously been treated with radiotherapy and, of those, recurrences were within the treated volume in 81%. It is therefore unlikely that our results are influenced by the inclusion of these patients as our results fit the previously reported results of other studies quite well.

References

1   Colorectal Cancer Collaborative Group: Adjuvant radiotherapy for rectal cancer: A systematic overview of 8507 patients from 22 randomised trials. Lancet 2001;358:1291–1304.
2   Camma C, Giunta M, Fiorica F, Pagliaro L, Craxi A, Cottone M: Preoperative radiotherapy for resectable rectal cancer. A meta-analysis. JAMA 2000;284:1008–1015.
3   Krook J, Moertel C, Gunderson L, Wieand H, Collins R, Beart R, Kubista T, Poon M, Meyers W, Mailliard J, Twito D, Morton R, Veeder M, Witzig T, Cha S, Vidyarthi S: Effective surgical adjuvant therapy for high risk rectal carcinoma. N Engl J Med 1991;324:709–715.
4   O'Connell M, Martenson J, Wieand H, Krook J, Macdonald J, Haller D, Mayer R, Gunderson L, Rich T: Improving adjuvant therapy for rectal cancer by combining protracted-infusion fluorouracil with radiation therapy after curative surgery. N Engl J Med 1994;331:502–507.
5   NIH Consensus Conference: Adjuvant therapy for patients with colon and rectal cancer. JAMA 1990;264:1444–1450.
6   Gastrointestinal Tumor Study Group: Prolongation of the disease free interval in surgically treated rectal carcinoma. N Engl J Med 1985;312:1465–1472.
7   Kapiteijn E, Marijnen C, Colenbrander A, Klein Kranenbarg E, Steup W, van Krieken J, van Houwelingen J, Leer J, van de Velde C: Local recurrence in patients with rectal cancer diagnosed between 1988 and 1992: A population-based study in the west Netherlands. Eur J Surg Oncol 1998;24:528–535.
8   Quirke P, Dixon M, Durdey P, Williams N: Local recurrence of rectal adenocarcinoma due to inadequate surgical resection. Histopathological study of lateral tumor spread and surgical excision. Lancet 1986;ii:996–999.
9   Hermanek P: Impact of surgeon's technique on outcome after treatment of rectal carcinoma. Dis Colon Rectum 1999;42:559–562.
10 MacFarlane J, Ryall R, Heald R: Mesorectal excision for rectal cancer. Lancet 1993;341:457–460.
11 Heald RJ, Ryall RD: Recurrence and survival after total mesorectal excision for rectal cancer. Lancet 1986;ii:1479–1482.
12 Gunderson L, Sosin H: Areas of failure found at reoperation (second or symptomatic look) following 'curative surgery' for adenocarcinoma of the rectum: Clinicopathologic correlation and implications for adjuvant therapy. Cancer 1974;34:1278–1292.

13   Pilipshen S, Heilweil M, Quan S, Sternberg S, Enker W: Patterns of pelvic recurrence following definitive resections of rectal cancer. Cancer 1984;53:1354–1362.

14   Wong C, Cummings B, Brierley J, Catton C, McLean M, Catton P, Hao Y: Treatment of locally recurrent rectal carcinoma – Results and prognostic factors. Int J Radiat Oncol Biol Phys 1998; 40:427–435.

15   Shoup M, Guillem J, Alektiar K, Liau K, Paty P, Cohen A, Wong WD, Minsky B: Predictors of survival in recurrent rectal cancer after resection and intraoperative radiotherapy. Dis Colon Rectum 2002;45:585–592.

16   Wanebo H, Koness J, Vezeridis M, Cohen S, Wrobleski D: Pelvic resection of recurrent rectal cancer. Ann Surg 1994;220:586–597.

17   Wiig J, Tveit K, Poulsen J, Olsen D, Giercksky K: Preoperative irradiation and surgery for recurrent rectal cancer: Will intraoperative radiotherapy (IORT) be of additional benefit? A prospective study. Radiother Oncol 2002;62:207–213.

18   Wolmark N, Wieand H, Hyams D, Colangelo L, Dimitrov N, Romond E, Wexler M, Prager D, Cruz A, Gordon P, Petrelli N, Deutsch M, Mamounas E, Wickerham D, Fisher E, Rockette H, Fisher B: Randomized trial of postoperative adjuvant chemotherapy with or without radiotherapy for carcinoma of the rectum: National Surgical Adjuvant Breast and Bowel Project Protocol R-02. J Natl Cancer Inst 2000;92:388–396.

19   Kapiteijn E, Marijnen C, Nagtegaal I, Putter H, Steup W, Wiggers T, Rutten H, Pahlman L, Glimelius B, van Krieken J, Leer J, van de Velde C: Preoperative radiotherapy combined with total mesorectal excision for resectable rectal cancer. N Engl J Med 2001;345:638–646.

20   Tepper J, O'Connell M, Niedzwiecki D, Hollis D, Benson A, Cummings B, Gunderson L, Macdonald J, Martenson J, Mayer R: Adjuvant therapy in rectal cancer: Analysis of stage, sex, and local control. Final report of Intergroup 0114. J Clin Oncol 2002;20:1744–1750.

21   McCall J, Cox M, Wattchow D: Analysis of local recurrence rates after surgery alone for rectal cancer. Int J Colorectal Dis 1995;10:126–132.

22   Gelber R, Goldhirsch A, Cole B, Wieand H, Schroeder G, Krook J: A quality-adjusted time without symptoms or toxicity (Q-TWiST) analysis of adjuvant radiation therapy and chemotherapy for resectable rectal cancer. J Natl Cancer Inst 1996;88:1039–1045.

23   Mak A, Rich T, Schultheiss T, Kavanagh B, Ota D, Romsdahl M: Late complications of postoperative radiation therapy for cancer of the rectum and rectosigmoid. Int J Radiat Oncol Biol Phys 1994;28:597–603.

24   Baglan K, Frazier R, Yan D, Huang R, Martinez A, Robertson J: The dose-volume relationship of acute small bowel toxicity from concurrent 5-FU-based chemotherapy and radiation therapy for rectal cancer. Int J Radiat Oncol Biol Phys 2002;52:176–183.

25   Letschert J, Lebesque J, Aleman B, Bosset J, Horiot J, Bartelink H, Cionini L, Hamers J, Leer J, van Glabbeke M: The volume effect in radiation-related small-bowel complications: Results of a clinical study of the EORTC Radiotherapy Cooperative Group in patients treated for rectal cancer. Radiother Oncol 1994;32:116–123.

26   Minsky B, Conti J, Huang Y, Knopf K: Relationship of acute gastrointestinal toxicity and volume of irradiated small bowel in patients receiving combined modality therapy for rectal cancer. J Clin Oncol 1995;13:1409–1416.

27   McDermott F, Hughes E, Pihl E, Johnson W, Price A: Local recurrence after potentially curative resection for rectal cancer in a series of 1008 patients. Br J Surg 1985;72:34–37.

28   Bagatzounis A, Kölbl O, Mueller G, Oppitz U, Willner J, Flentje M: Das lokoregionäre Rezidiv des Rektumkarzinoms. Eine comutertomographische Analyse und ein Zielvolumenkonzept für die adjuvante Radiotherapie. Strahlenther Onkol 1997;173:68–75.

29   Galandiuk S, Wieand H, Moertel C, Cha S, Fitzgibbons R, Pemberton J, Wolff B: Patterns of recurrence after curative resection of carcinoma of the colon and rectum. Surg Gynecol Obstet 1992;174:27–32.

30   Hoffman JP, Riley L, Carp N, Litwin S: Isolated locally recurrent rectal cancer: A review of incidence, presentation, and management. Semin Oncol 1993;20:506–519.

31   Mendenhall W, Million R, Pfaff W: Patterns of recurrence in adenocarcinoma of the rectum and rectosigmoid treated with surgery alone: Implications in treatment planning with adjuvant radiation therapy. Int J Radiat Oncol Biol Phys 1983;9:977–985.

32   Wiig J, Wolff P, Tveit K, Giercksky K: Location of pelvic recurrence after 'curative' low anterior resection for rectal cancer. Eur J Surg Oncol 1999;25:590–594.
33   Höcht S, Wiegel T, Hammad R, Hinkelbein W: Pelvic sites of recurrence in rectal cancer. Lancet 2002;360:879–880.

Dr. Stefan Höcht
Klinik für Radioonkologie und Strahlentherapie
Charité, Campus Benjamin Franklin
Hindenburgdamm 30, DE–12200 Berlin (Germany)
Tel. +49 30 8445 3058, Fax +49 30 8445 2991, E-Mail stefan.hoecht@medizin.fu-berlin.de

Wiegel T, Höcht S, Sternemann M, Buhr HJ, Hinkelbein W (eds): Controversies in Gastrointestinal Tumor Therapy. Front Radiat Ther Oncol. Basel, Karger, 2004, vol 38, pp 52–56

....

Intraoperative Radiotherapy – Special Focus: Recurrent Rectal Carcinoma

M. Treiber[a], T. Lehnert[b], S. Oertel[a], R. Krempien[a], M. Bischof[a], M. Buechler[b], M. Wannenmacher[a], J. Debus[a]

Departments of [a]Clinical Radiology and [b]Surgery, University of Heidelberg, Heidelberg, Germany

Rectal cancer has a high rate of local recurrences and still has a poor prognosis. Surgical abilities are limited due to the involvement of bone, vascular or visceral structures, and curative treatment is possible in less than 10%. Palliative strategies are aimed to prevent the debilitating symptoms of pelvic failures. Intraoperative radiotherapy (IORT) gives the possibility of a locally restricted dose escalation [1]. In addition, for previously irradiated patients, IORT often offers the last chance for additional high-dose radiation [2]. In our department we established multimodal treatment including surgery, IORT and external beam radiotherapy (EBRT) to improve local control and prevent symptoms of pelvic failures.

Materials and Methods

From August 1991 to December 2001, 65 patients (31 males and 34 females) with recurrent rectal carcinomas underwent surgery with IORT. The mean patient age was 59 years. All patients had extensive preoperative evaluations, including CT scans of the abdomen and pelvis. Failure locations were at the anastomosis (n = 24), the presacrum (n = 26) and the pelvic side wall (n = 15). At the time of failure diagnosis 21 patients showed lymph node involvement and 13 patients had distant metastases (12 in the liver and 1 in the lungs).

All operations were performed with the intent of complete resection. Complete resection (R0) was possible in 29 patients, 17 patients had microscopic (R1) and 19 patients had macroscopic (R2) tumor residuals. 18 patients had an anterior resection, 30 patients had

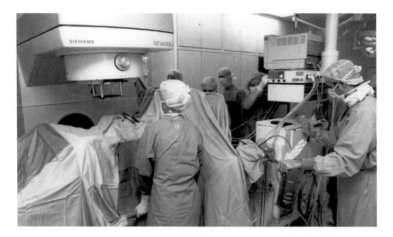

Fig. 1. Typical IORT situation. After tumor resection the applicator has been placed and fixed by special equipment. Then the patient is placed under the accelerator. The entire IORT procedure (including positioning, irradiation and replacing) required 20 min.

an abdominoperineal resection and only local resection was possible in 17 patients. The type of surgical procedure was determined by the extent and location of the tumor and the nature of prior surgery.

Intraoperative electron-beam irradiation was performed with a dedicated facility (Siemens Mevatron ME; fig. 1). The small bowel was covered with a moist towel and placed cranially in the irradiation field. Both ureters were safely placed outside the IORT field in all patients. Beams were shaped by circular chrome-plated brass applicators. The applicator diameters varied from 5 to 12 (mean 7.5) cm. Beam alignment was achieved with an air-docking system guided by an arrangement of laser beams within the gantry (fig. 2). Electron-beam IORT was prescribed to the 90% isodose. A mean IORT dose of 12.5 (10–20) Gy was delivered at a dose rate of 9 Gy/min.

54 patients had an additional 3D-planned EBRT with a total dose of 41.4 (single dose 1.8) Gy, either preoperatively (n = 36) or postoperatively (n = 18). Simultaneous chemotherapy (5-FU/leucovorin) was given in 46 patients, which consisted of bolus intravenous leucovorin (200 mg/m^2) and intravenous bolus fluorouracil (400 mg/m^2) in weeks 1 and 4 of EBRT.

Results

After a median follow-up of 36 months and a minimum follow-up of 2 years, a second local failure was observed in 15 patients, resulting in a local control rate of 68%. The failure location was evaluated with CT scans and correlated with the IORT and EBRT field margins (IORT fields were clip-marked

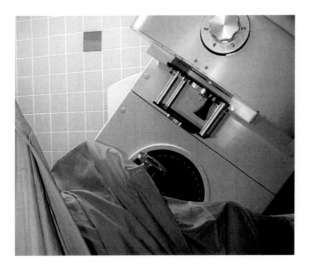

Fig. 2. The accelerator is adjusted to the applicator with an air-docking laser system.

if they were not at the presacral area, e.g. pelvic side-wall). Five recurrences were within the IORT treatment field (7.7%) and 6 at the IORT field margin within the EBRT field. In additional 4 anastomotic re-recurrences were seen. As expected the presence of residual disease at the time of IORT had a negative impact on local tumor control. The actuarial 5-year local control probability was 78% in patients with complete resection and 58% in patients with microscopic residues. These local control rates were significantly higher compared to patients with macroscopic residues (29%). There was no statistical difference between R0 and R1 resected patients.

Sufficient pain relief was reported by all patients within 10 days after surgery and IORT.

The median disease-free interval was 11.9 months. Distant metastases were found in 30 patients (12 patients with local failure, alone in 18 patients). The 5-year overall survival rate was low (39%) due to the high distant metastasis rate. 17 patients died due to progressive disease, and 1 patient died of other causes.

Most patients tolerated the treatment well. We had no perioperative mortality (within 30 days after surgery). Perioperative morbidity (like dehiscence or abscess) was not increased. 3 patients developed ureter stenosis as a long-term complication, but in none of the patients were the ureters inside the IORT field. Neuropathy was not observed. Acute and late toxicities were not increased by the combined treatment with surgery, IORT and EBRT, compared to surgery and EBRT alone.

Discussion

Curative resection of recurrences from rectal carcinoma confined to the pelvis could be performed only in some selected situations, such as anastomotic-limited recurrences, or after early detection. Attempts to increase surgical radicality enhance perioperative morbidity and mortality. Higher doses of irradiation in the preoperative or postoperative course increase the probability of local tumor control, but in the same way perioperative morbidity is increased too. IORT allows the delivery of a high single dose to a sharply delineated volume, while sparing normal adjacent tissues.

In the last years some studies on IORT in recurrent rectal carcinoma have been published [1–6]. The best results were shown if complete resection had been possible. The local control rates after IORT were increased compared to surgery and EBRT alone, as in our patients. There was also a benefit for patients treated with IORT after R1 resection in our study. We could show that the local control rate of these patients was 58%. There was no significant difference compared to patients with complete resection.

In the literature no information was given on the ratio of in-field IORT versus out-field failures. In our study failure locations were inside the IORT field in only 5 patients (7.7%).

The risk of side effects is increased by high additional EBRT doses (50.4–54.4 Gy) as described in former studies [7]. We could show that there are no IORT-related complications if both ureters are safely placed outside the IORT field and moderate doses of EBRT (in combination with chemotherapy) are applied.

In the patient series treated at the Ullevaal Hospital Oslo, Norway, the R0/R1-stage patients survived significantly longer than the R2 group [6]. We could see a trend to better survival in R0/R1-resected patients, but the difference was not significant. The overall survival is bad for macroscopic incompletely resected patients due to their high rate of distant metastases.

Conclusion

We conclude that IORT is a feasible and safe technique for patients with recurrent rectal carcinoma. Local control in recurrent rectal carcinomas appears to be improved in this series. IORT offers a locally restricted dose escalation by optimal normal tissue sparing. Palliation, especially pain relief, was achieved in all our patients and is an important effect of IORT. The benefit of IORT for overall survival has to be proven in larger trials.

References

1   Merrick HW, Crucitti A, Padgett BJ, Dobelbower RR Jr: IORT as a surgical adjuvant for pelvic recurrence of rectal cancer; in Vaeth JM (ed): Intraoperative Radiation Therapy in the Treatment of Cancer. 6th IORT Symposium and 31st San Francisco Cancer Symposium, San Francisco, 1996. Front Radiat Ther Oncol. Basel, Karger, 1997, vol 31, pp 234–237.

2   Haddock MG, Gunderson LL, Nelson H, Cha S, Devine RM, Dozois RR, Wolff BG: Intraoperative irradiation for locally recurrent colorectal cancer in previously irradiated patients; in Vaeth JM (ed): Intraoperative Radiation Therapy in the Treatment of Cancer. 6th IORT Symposium and 31st San Francisco Cancer Symposium, San Francisco, 1996. Front Radiat Ther Oncol. Basel, Karger, 1997, vol 31, pp 243–244.

3   Bussères E, Gilly FN, Rouanet P, Mahe MA, Roussel A, Delannes M, Gerard JP, Dubois JB, Richaud P: Recurrences of rectal cancers: Results of a multimodal approach with intraoperative radiation therapy. Int J Radiat Oncol Biol Phys 1996;34:49–56.

4   Martinez-Monge R, Jurado M, Azinovic I, Aristu J, Fernandez-Hidalgo O, Lopez G, Calvo FA: Preoperative chemoradiation and adjuvant surgery in locally advanced or recurrent cervical carcinoma. Rev Med Univ Navarra 1997;41:19–26.

5   Lindel K, Willett CG, Shellito PC, Ott MJ, Clark J, Grossbard M, Ryan D, Ancukiewicz M: Intraoperative radiation therapy for locally advanced recurrent rectal or rectosigmoid cancer. Radiother Oncol 2001;58:83–87.

6   Wiig JN, Tveit KM, Poulsen JP, Olsen DR, Giercksky KE: Preoperative irradiation and surgery for recurrent rectal cancer. Will intraoperative radiotherapy (IORT) be of additional benefit? A prospective study. Radiother Oncol 2002;62:207–213.

7   Gunderson LL, Nelson H, Martenson JA, Cha S, Haddock M, Devine R, Fieck JM, Wolff B, Dozois R, O'Connell MJ: Intraoperative electron end external beam irradiation with or without 5-fluorouracil and maximum surgical resection for previously unirradiated, locally recurrence colorectal cancer. Dis Col Rectum 1996;39:1379–1395.

Dr. Martina Treiber
Klinik Radiologie, Universität Heidelberg
Kopfklinik, INF 400
DE–69120 Heidelberg (Germany)
Tel. +49 6221/56 8201, Fax +49 6221/56 5353,
E-Mail martina_treiber@med.uni-heidelberg.de

Wiegel T, Höcht S, Sternemann M, Buhr HJ, Hinkelbein W (eds): Controversies in Gastrointestinal
Tumor Therapy. Front Radiat Ther Oncol. Basel, Karger, 2004, vol 38, pp 57–66

....

Local Recurrence of Rectal Carcinoma: Radio-Oncologic Strategies

P.H. Lukas

Universitätsklinik für Strahlentherapie, Radioonkologie,
Medizinische Universität Innsbruck, Innsbruck, Oesterreich

Looking for radio-oncologic strategies concerning the local recurrence of rectal carcinoma, a systematic review of the literature was recently undertaken by Wong et al. [1] to address the question: what is the most effective dose fractionation schedule for the relief of symptoms in patients with pelvic recurrence from rectal or colorectal carcinoma? The authors came to the following result: 'The optimal dose fractionation schedule for the palliation of pelvic recurrence from rectal carcinoma remains undefined. Well-designed randomized studies, with study arms that are sufficiently diverse biologically to allow the detection of a dose-response relationship, if one existed, equipped with suitable symptom control end points, are necessary to provide a clinically relevant answer' [1].

However, there are some hints on how to deal with the problem regarding history and status of the patient as well as primarily applied treatment modalities.

In general the following parameters influence the outcome of a second treatment in rectal cancer: 'Upon multivariate analysis, overall survival was positively correlated with ECOG performance status (p = 0.0001), absence of extrapelvic metastases (p = 0.0001), long intervals from initial surgery to radiation therapy for local recurrence (p = 0.0001), total radiation dose (p = 0.0001), and absence of obstructive uropathy (p = 0.0013). Pelvic disease progression-free rates were positively correlated with ECOG performance status (p = 0.0001), total radiation dose (p = 0.0001), and previous conservative surgery for the primary (p = 0.02)' [2].

There are a number of relevant options involving radiotherapy in the treatment of rectal local recurrences: (1) conventional external beam radiotherapy (EBRT) with or without concomitant chemotherapy, administered pre- or postoperatively; (2) intensity-modulated radiotherapy (IMRT) or other high precision

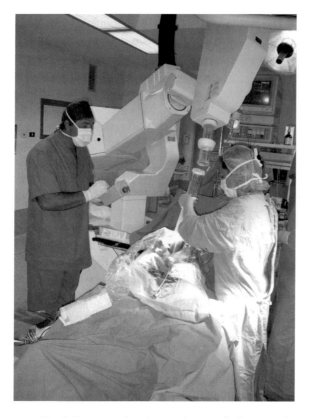

Fig. 2. Intraoperative electron beam radiotherapy using a mobile linear accelerator.

radical surgery and intraoperative IORT boost: 'Fifteen patients received a radical resection (R0), 8 a microscopic non-radical resection (R1), and 14 a macroscopic non-radical resection (R2). The overall 3-year local control (LC), disease-free survival (DFS), and overall survival rates were 60, 32, and 58%, respectively. Radicality of resection (R0/R1 vs. R2) turned out to be the significant factor for improved survival ($p < 0.05$), DFS ($p = 0.0008$), and LC ($p = 0.01$). Preoperative (re-)irradiation is the other significant factor in survival ($p = 0.005$) and DFS ($p = 0.001$) and was almost significant for LC ($p = 0.08$). After external beam radiation therapy (EBRT) a significantly higher resection rate was obtained (R0/R1 vs. R2 $p = 0.001$)'.

In an update in 2001 the same group compared primarily non-resectable rectal carcinoma with local recurrence, using EBRT and IORT and came to the following results: 'After 3 years, the local control, disease-free survival and survival rates for the locally advanced primary rectal cancer group were 74, 60 and 55%, respectively, and for the locally recurrent rectal cancer group 64, 34 and 50% respectively' [8].

Also in terms of quality of life the outcome was comparable between both groups: '56 and 63% respectively had been able to resume employment, 53 and 59% respectively had been able to resume their previous lifestyle, 15 and 27% respectively indicated radicular pain as a new symptom, 26 and 46% respectively stated problems with walking, 42 and 44% respectively stated problems with urinating and 59 and 52% respectively a reduction in sexual activity' [8].

Intraoperative HDR-Brachytherapy

Concerning the technique of IORT results seem to be comparable using either electron beam or HDR brachytherapy. Harrison et al. [9] published data on 22 patients with primary unresectable disease and 46 patients who presented with recurrent disease: 'In general, the patients with primary unresectable disease received preoperative chemotherapy with 5-fluorouracil (5-FU) and leucovorin, and external beam irradiation to 4,500–5,040 cGy, followed by surgical resection and HDR-IORT (1,000–2,000 cGy). In general, the patients with recurrent disease were treated with surgical resection and HDR-IORT (1,000–2,000 cGy) alone. For patients with recurrent disease, the 2-year actuarial local control rate was 63%. The disease-free survival was 47% (71% for negative margins and 0% for positive margins; p = 0.04)'. As already stated, the last figures mean that IORT alone might not be sufficient and EBRT has to be added whenever possible.

In our own experience after a median follow up of 19 months overall survival was 56% in patients with negative margins against 49% in patients with R1+R2+Rx resection. This can be interpreted in a way that the intraoperative boost might be able to equalize the disadvantage of R1 or even R2 resections when the rest of the tumor layer, as in our series, does not exceed 3 mm of thickness. Unfortunately this might never be proven as all attempts to evaluate this matter in randomized trials failed due to the small number of patients for accrual (fig. 3, 4).

Hyperthermia

A number of other modalities combined with radiotherapy are still under investigation. One which is of increasing interest is hyperthermia. Some

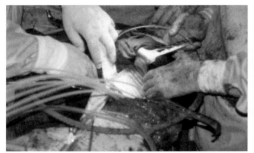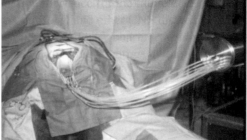

Fig. 3. Intraoperative HDR-brachytherapy using the Munich flab method.

publications [19, 20] indicate a possible advantage for combining hyperthermia with chemoradiation against chemoradiation alone, but until now this could not be proven for rectal carcinoma in randomized trials.

Radiotherapy Combined with Intra-Arterial Chemotherapy

Another method, not used in rectal carcinoma alone, is the combination with intra-arterially applied chemotherapy [21]. An especially developed technique is necessary to avoid serious side effects, which might be responsible for the missing evaluation of the method in further series.

High LET Radiation

Other modalities are under investigation. Proton therapy or other high LET radiation is a powerful tool to increase dose in tumor tissue. In his Gray lecture 2001 Suit [10] stated: 'The technology of RT is clearly experiencing intense and rapid technical developments as pertains to treatment planning and dose delivery. It is predicted that radical dose RT will move to proton beam technology and that the treatment will be four dimensional'. But these methods are very expensive and will therefore not be available everywhere in the near future (fig. 5).

Variations in Fractionation

Variations in fractionation schedules have also been investigated for the treatment of rectal carcinoma. Hyperfractionation and acceleration are useful for the shortening of treatment time in palliative modalities.

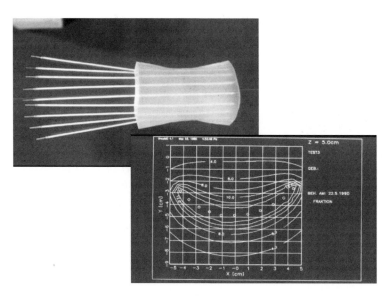

Fig. 4. The mobile and flexible flab and its dose distribution on the surface and in a depth of 4 cm.

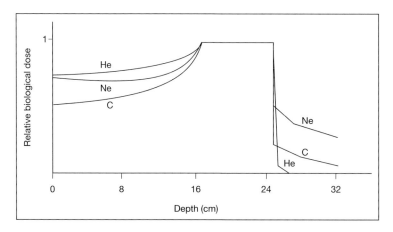

Fig. 5. Relative biological dose depth curve of different ions. Variations in fractionation.

Glynne-Jones et al. [11] experienced a good effect on quality of life in rectal recurrence: 'A total dose of 54 Gy was given in 36 fractions over 12 consecutive days; three fractions of 1.5 Gy were employed each day with an interfraction interval of 6 h. Of these 19 patients, 13 had local pelvic recurrence from rectal carcinoma. Complete pain relief was achieved in recurrent rectal cancer in 100% of patients, at a median of 15 days since commencing radiotherapy (range 7–63 days), and has been maintained for mean and median durations of 19 and 18 months respectively (range 1.5–45 months)'.

Combination with New Agents

Last but not least the combination with new agents, especially those with radiosensitizing effects, is of growing interest. As we learned from the experience with gemcitabine, new drugs should be tested for their radiosensitizing capabilities early in preclinical studies before being implemented into clinical routine by internal oncologists in order to prevent patients from increased toxicities in combing these new drugs with conventional fractionated radiotherapy. If this is taken into account, 'further improvement in response and - survival could be achieved by using novel chemotherapeutic agents or through tumor-selective molecular targeting strategies that enhance the effects of chemotherapy, radiotherapy, or both. Irinotecan (CPT-11, Camptosar) is a novel chemotherapy agent being evaluated clinically as a radiosensitizing agent in rectal cancer. Inhibition of several molecular targets-such as epidermal growth factor receptor, ras oncogene activation, the cyclooxygenase-2 (COX-2) enzyme, and neoangiogenesis-appears to be tumor-selective in preclinical models. COX-2 expression has been shown to enhance cytotoxic therapy in preclinical models. In vitro and in vivo studies show that selective COX-2 inhibition enhances the effects of radiotherapy as well as chemotherapy' [12].

Conclusion

There are numerous ways to re-treat patients with local recurrence of rectal carcinoma. The chosen treatment should carefully be harmonized with the primarily applied modalities and the history and status of the patient. Curative results can be achieved under favorable circumstances, as well as reasonable palliation in progressive or metastatic disease. New treatment modalities have to be proven carefully.

References

1   Wong R, Thomas G, Cummings B, Froud P, Shelley W, Withers R, Williams J: In search of a dose-response relationship with radiotherapy in the management of recurrent rectal carcinoma in the pelvis: A systematic review. Int J Radiat Oncol Biol Phys 1998;40:437–446.

2   Wong CS, Cummings BJ, Brierley JD, Catton CN, McLean M, Catton P, Hao Y: Treatment of locally recurrent rectal carcinoma – Results and prognostic factors. Int J Radiat Oncol Phys 1998; 40:427–435.

3   National Cancer Institute (NCI). March 13, 1991 (http://www.nlm.nih.gov/databases/alerts/rectal_cancer.html)

4   Martling A, Holm T, Johansson H, Rutqvist LE, Cedermark B, Stockholm Colorectal Cancer Study Group: The Stockholm II trial on preoperative radiotherapy in rectal carcinoma: Long-term follow-up of a population-based study. Cancer 2001;92:896–902.

5   Bagatzounis A, Kolbl O, Muller G, Oppitz U, Willner J, Flentje M: The locoregional recurrence of rectal carcinoma. A computed tomographic analysis and a target volume concept for adjuvant radiotherapy. Strahlenther Onkol 1997;173:68–75.

6   Gunderson LL: Indications for and results of combined modality treatment of colorectal cancer. Acta Oncol 1999;38:7–21.

7   Mannaerts GH, Martijn H, Crommelin MA, Stultiens GN, Dries W, van Driel OJ, Rutten HJ: Intraoperative electron beam radiation therapy for locally recurrent rectal carcinoma. Int J Radiat Oncol Biol Phys 1999;45:297–308.

8   Mannaerts GH, Martijn H, Rutten HJ, Hanssens PE, Wiggers T: Local tumor control and (disease-free) survival after surgery with pre- and intraoperative radiotherapy for primary non-resectable rectal carcinoma and local recurrence. Ned Tijdschr Geneeskd 2001;145: 1460–1466.

9   Harrison LB, Minsky BD, Enker WE, Mychalczak B, Guillem J, Paty PB, Anderson L, White C, Cohen AM: High dose rate intraoperative radiation therapy (HDR-IORT) as part of the management strategy for locally advanced primary and recurrent rectal cancer. Int J Radiat Oncol Biol Phys 1998;42:325–330.

10 Suit H: The Gray Lecture 2001: Coming technical advances in radiation oncology. Int J Radiat Oncol Biol Phys 2002;53:798–809.

11 Glynne-Jones R, Saunders MI, Hoskin P, Phillips H: A pilot study of continuous, hyperfractionated, accelerated radiotherapy in rectal adenocarcinoma. Clin Oncol (R Coll Radiol) 1999;11: 334–339.

12 Crane CH, Janjan NA, Mason K, Milas L: Preoperative chemoradiation for locally advanced rectal cancer: Emerging treatment strategies. Oncology (Huntingt) 2002;16(suppl 5): 39–44.

13 Lokich JJ, Ahlgreen JD, Gullo JJ, et al: A prospective randomized comparison of continuous infusion fluorouracil with a conventional bolus schedule in metastatic colorectal carcinoma: Mid-Atlantic Oncology Program Study. J Clin Oncol 1989;7:425–432.

14 O'Conell M, Martenson J, Rich T, et al: Protracted venous infusion (PVI) 5-fluorouracil (5-FU) as a component of effective combined modality postoperative surgical adjuvant therapy for high-risk rectal cancer. Soc Clin Oncol 1993;12:193.

15 Rich TA, Skibber JM, Ajani JA, et al: Preoperative infusional chemoradiation therapy for stage T3 rectal cancer. Int J Radiat Oncol Biol Phys 1995;32:1025–1029.

16 Eble MJ, Lehnert T, Treiber M, Latz D, Herfarth C, Wannenmacher M: Moderate dose intraoperative and external beam radiotherapy for locally recurrent rectal carcinoma. Radiother Oncol 1998;49:169–174.

17 Nag S, Martinez-Monge R, Martin EW: Intraoperative electron beam radiotherapy in recurrent colorectal carcinoma. J Surg Oncol 1999;72:66–71.

18 Lindel K, Willett CG, Shellito PC, Ott MJ, Clark J, Grossbard M, Ryan D, Ancukiewicz M: Intraoperative radiation therapy for locally advanced recurrent rectal or rectosigmoid cancer. Radiother Oncol 2001;58:83–87.

19 Wust P, Gellermann J, Rau B, Loffel J, Speidel A, Stahl H, Riess H, Vogl TJ, Felix R, Schlag PM: Hyperthermia in the multimodal therapy of advanced rectal carcinomas. Recent Res Cancer Res 1996;142:281–309.

20 Rau B, Wust P, Riess H, Schlag PM: Radiochemotherapy plus hyperthermia in rectal carcinoma. Schweiz Rundsch Med Prax 2001;90:587–592.

Local Recurrence of Rectal Carcinoma: Radio-Oncologic Strategies

21 Knysh VI, Kim FP, Goldobenko GV, Tsariuk VF, Barsukov IuA: Definition, classification and combined treatment of locally invasive rectal neoplasms (in Russian). Khirurgiia (Mosk) 1994; 10:20–23.

O. Univ.-Prof. Dr. med. P.H. Lukas
Universitäts-Klinik für Strahlentherapie – Radioonkologie
Leopold-Franzens-Universität Innsbruck
Anichstrasse 35, AT–6020 Innsbruck (Austria)
Tel. +43 512 504 2800, Fax +43 512 504 2869, E-Mail peter.lukas@uibk.ac.at

Wiegel T, Höcht S, Sternemann M, Buhr HJ, Hinkelbein W (eds): Controversies in Gastrointestinal
Tumor Therapy. Front Radiat Ther Oncol. Basel, Karger, 2004, vol 38, pp 67–75

....

Diagnostic Imaging of Pancreatic Cancer – The Role of PET

Michael Zimny

Department of Nuclear Medicine, University Hospital, Aachen, Germany

Adenocarcinoma of the pancreas is among the most frequent causes of cancer-related deaths in patients with gastrointestinal malignances. Curative therapy is restricted to patients with limited and resectable disease. However, late onset of often unspecific symptoms explains that the majority of patients present with advanced and non-resectable disease at primary diagnosis. Thus, the overall 5-year survival rate for pancreatic cancer is below 1–5% [1, 2]. However, even in resectable tumors the 5-year survival is only 5–15% [3–5] indicating that pancreatoduodenectomy represents a palliative procedure for the majority of patients with pancreatic cancer [6].

Despite a battery of imaging tools and recent advances in computed tomography (CT) and magnetic resonance imaging (MRI), the differential diagnosis of pancreatic adenocarcinoma and chronic focal pancreatitis is still a challenge [7]. Since the early 1990s positron emission tomography (PET) with the radiolabeled glucose analog 2-[^{18}F]-fluoro-2-deoxy-*D*-glucose (FDG PET) has been used in oncology. The feasibility of visualizing malignant tumors with FDG PET is based on the early observation of Warburg et al. [8] that the malignant transformation of cells is accompanied by an increased glycolytic rate. For both, FDG and glucose, the transport into the cell is facilitated by glucose transport proteins (GLUT). Among other malignant tumors, an increased expression of GLUT has been reported for pancreatic cancer [9, 10]. Like glucose, FDG is phosphorylated by the hexokinase-mediated reaction. However, the next steps in the biochemical pathway of glucose are blocked for FDG and, hence, FDG accumulates in the cell in relation to glucose consumption. Absolute measurements of regional radioactivity concentrations enable the quantitative or semi-quantitative assessment of parameters of regional glucose metabolism, e.g. the

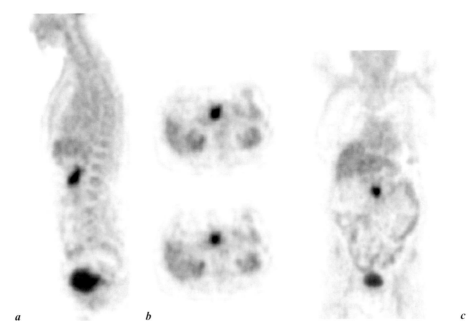

a   *b*   *c*

Fig. 1. Sagittal (***a***), transversal (***b***), and coronal (***c***) slices showing intensive and focal FDG uptake in the head of the pancreas in a patient with adenocarcinoma of the pancreas.

metabolic rate for glucose, the transport rate for FDG, or the standardized uptake value. A number of studies, recently summarized by Gambhir et al. [11], described encouraging results for FDG PET for the primary diagnosis, staging and therapy monitoring of a variety of malignant diseases including pancreatic cancer.

The early studies of FDG PET in pancreatic cancer focused on the differential diagnosis of pancreatic masses [12, 13]. A typical example of pancreatic adenocarcinoma with intense and focal FDG uptake is shown in figure 1. A pilot study by Bares et al. [13] reported a high detection rate of pancreatic cancer with FDG PET. These encouraging results were confirmed later on in a larger series of patients with a sensitivity of 85% and a specificity of 84% [14]. In this study all but 1 false-negative findings occurred in hyperglycemic patients. Thus, the sensitivity improved to 98% if hyperglycemic patients were excluded. False-positive findings were observed in patients with active chronic pancreatitis. Similar results were reported by Diederichs et al. [15]. To date a number of studies with more than 900 patients have been published (table 1). The median sensitivity, specificity, negative predictive value, positive predictive value, and accuracy were 93, 83, 81, 92, and 87%, respectively.

Table 1. Summary of the results of FDG PET for the differentiation of pancreatic lesions

Author	n	Sensitivity, %	Specificity, %	Prevalence[1], %
Bares et al. [39][a], 1994	40	93	85	68
Stollfuss et al. [40][2, b], 1995	73	95	90	59
Friess et al. [41][b], 1995	80	94	88	60
Inokuma et al. [42], 1995	46	94	82	76
Kato et al. [43], 1995	24	93	78	63
Bares et al. [44][a], 1996	85	85	77	65
Ho et al. [45], 1996	14	(8/8)	(4/6)	
Zimny et al. [14][a], 1997	106	85	84	70
	72[3]	98	85	65
Diederichs et al. [15][b], 1998	152	86	78	68
Keogan et al. [46], 1998	37	88	83	68
Rajput et al. [47], 1998	15	89	100	82
Sendler et al. [48][c], 1998	46	86	67	61
Delbeke et al, [49][2, d], 1999	65	92	85	80
Rose et al. [25][d], 1999	65	92	85	80
Imdahl et al. [21][2, e], 1999	48	96	100	56
Diederichs et al. [18][b], 1999	304[4]	81	82	52
Sendler et al. [27][c], 2000	42	71	64	74
Nakamoto et al. [22][2], 2000	47	96[5]	75	57
		100[6]	80	
Koyama et al. [50], 2001	86	82	81	76
Sperti et al. [26], 2001	55	94	97	31
Nitzsche et al. [23][7, e], 2002	15	100	100	44
Papos et al. [51], 2001	22	100	88	27
Sum[8]	907			
Range[8]	11–304	71–100	64–100	27–82
Median[8]	47	93	83	66

[1]Prevalence of pancreatic carcinoma.

[2]Diagnosis based on standardized uptake values (SUV).

[3]Subgroup of patients with normal blood glucose levels (<6.2 mmol/l).

[4]132 malignant tumors of the pancreas, including 91 cases of ductal adenocarcinoma and 16 cases of ampullary carcinoma.

[5]SUV 1 h after FDG i.v.

[6]SUV 2 h after FDG i.v. combined with retention index.

[7]Diagnosis based on time activity curves derived from kinetic data.

[8]Pooled data including only results of the publications with the largest series of patients of each institution.

[a–e]Publications from the same institute.

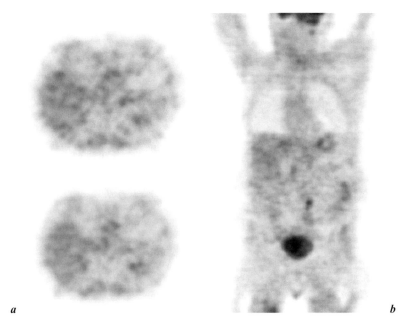

a   *b*

Fig. 2. Transversal (*a*) and coronal (*b*) slices of a patient with chronic pancreatitis showing only moderate and diffuse FDG uptake in the pancreas.

However, there is a broad range of results for sensitivity (71–100%) and specificity (64–100%). This can be mainly attributed to different patient selection criteria including the prevalence of pancreatic cancer and patients with diabetes as well as the prevalence of active chronic pancreatitis.

Especially Shreve [16] observed a considerable number of false-positive PET findings in patients with inflammatory processes of the pancreas. Intense and even focal FDG uptake of inflammatory processes is a known phenomenon and related to a high glucose metabolism of macrophages [17]. This is especially relevant in acute and active chronic pancreatitis. Diederichs et al. [18] showed in a large series of patients that the specificity of FDP PET to differentiate pancreatic cancer and chronic pancreatitis was related to the level of the C-reactive protein. In patients with a C-reactive protein concentration of >10 ng/ml the specificity of FDG PET was only 40% compared to 87% if the concentration of the C-reactive protein was <10 ng/ml. However, in non-active chronic pancreatitis the content of inflammatory cells is limited and, furthermore, the expression of the GLUT1 is low. Thus, the FDG uptake of the pancreas in the majority of patients with chronic pancreatitis is low (fig. 2) [10].

Recently, several authors recommended modifications to the acquisition protocol to improve the specificity of FDG PET. Based on observations of Hamberg et al. [19] and Hustinx et al. [20] that the FDG uptake of malignant tumors reaches a plateau as late as 2 h after intravenous administration of FDG and that benign lesions are more likely to show a decrease of the FDG uptake in this time period, Imdahl et al. [21] and Nakamoto et al. [22] showed that later acquisition or acquisitions at two different time points may improve the specificity of FDG PET. With the assessment of the FDG uptake of a lesion of the pancreas after 60 and 120 min the diagnostic accuracy to differentiate pancreatic cancer and chronic pancreatitis improved to 92 compared to 83% for the standard acquisition at 60 min after FDG administration [22]. There is evidence that time-activity curves of the FDG uptake derived from dynamic PET studies may further improve the differentiation of benign and malignant lesions of the pancreas [23].

Several authors compared the diagnostic accuracy of FDG PET with other imaging modalities. Diederichs et al. [24] reported the results of a receiver operating curves analysis (ROC) of FDG PET, CT, and endoscopic retrograde cholangiopancreatography (ERCP) in 159 patients. With an optimal area under the curve of 1.0, i.e. a diagnostic accuracy of 100%, the values were 0.82 for PET, 0.93 for ERCP, and 0.82 for CT. The combination of ERCP and PET further improved the diagnostic accuracy with an area under the curve of 0.95. In a subgroup of euglycemic patients with normal C-reactive protein levels the areas under the curves were 0.92, 0.94, 0.82 for PET, ERCP, and CT, respectively. Interestingly, the accuracy of PET was 84% in 54 patients with indeterminate CT and/or ERCP studies. There is further evidence that FDG PET is superior to helical CT for the differential diagnosis of pancreatic lesions [21, 25, 26]. Imdahl et al. [21] and Rose et al. [25] reported a significantly higher diagnostic accuracy for PET (97 and 91%) compared to CT (80 and 65%). Sperti et al. [26] focused on the diagnosis of cystic lesions of the pancreas. Again FDG PET was superior to CT with a sensitivity of 94 versus 65% and a specificity of 97 and 87%, respectively. In contrast, Sendler et al. [27] reported disappointing results for both helical CT (accuracy 68%) and FDG PET (accuracy 69%).

So far, a small number of studies have addressed the accuracy of FDG PET for the diagnosis of liver metastases or lymph node metastases [28, 29]. Fröhlich et al. [28] reported a sensitivity of 97% for the detection of liver metastases >1 cm. However, the detection rate was significantly affected by the size of the metastases resulting in an overall sensitivity of 67%. The value of FDG PET – as well as any other noninvasive imaging modality – for the preoperative staging of lymph node metastases is limited. In 36 patients with pancreatic cancer who underwent lymph node resection the sensitivity of PET was 50% (specificity 70%; own unpublished data). The sensitivity was affected by a high proportion of microscopic lymph node metastases. These results have recently been confirmed by Diederichs et al. [24].

Because of the fact that FDG PET is predominately a functional imaging modality that provides only little morphological information, it is obvious that PET cannot replace morphological imaging for the assessment of local tumor spread or resectability. On the contrary, a combination of morphological and functional imaging using either the fusion of image data that were obtained with independent imaging devices [30–32] or image data of recently introduced combined PET/CT [33] may be the ideal approach to describe pancreatic tumors with respect to morphological parameters (e.g. size, relationship to surrounding tissues and structures) or functional characteristics of pancreatic tumors like the glucose metabolism.

Besides the preoperative diagnosis and staging of pancreatic masses there is evidence that with the semiquantitative assessment of glucose metabolism, FDG PET provides prognostic information in patients with pancreatic cancer. In a small group of 14 patients Nakata et al. [34] showed that a high FDG uptake of pancreatic cancer was related to a significantly shorter survival time than a low FDG uptake. Based on an evaluation of 52 patients with pancreatic cancer, Zimny et al. [35] reported a median survival time of only 5 months in patients with an intense FDG uptake compared to 9 months in patients with a moderately increased glucose metabolism. A multivariate analysis including also the stage of disease and the tumor marker Ca 19–9 showed that the FDG uptake was an independent factor of prognosis [35]. These results were later on confirmed by Nakata et al. [36].

Recently, FDG PET performed before and after chemotherapy or radio-therapy has been used to assess the treatment response. Maisey et al. [37] performed FDG PET before and 1 month after chemotherapy and observed a significantly shorter survival time in patients with residual FDG uptake after chemotherapy. Higashi et al. [38] observed that serial PET scans were superior to serial CT scans to assess the response of pancreatic cancer to intraoperative radiotherapy.

In conclusion, the diagnostic accuracy of FDG PET to differentiate pancreatic masses is very similar to the results of modern morphological imaging tools. FDG PET represents a complementary imaging procedure if morphological imaging is indeterminate. One of the shortcomings of FDG PET is the lack of sufficient morphological information for the assessment of local resectability. Thus, a combination of PET and CT or MRI may become the method of choice for a comprehensive preoperative staging of pancreatic cancer. Furthermore, the assessment of the glucose metabolism of pancreatic cancer with FDG PET reveals relevant prognostic information and, perhaps of more importance, allows early assessment of treatment response.

References

1   Bakkevold KE, Kambestad B: Long-term survival following radical and palliative treatment of patients with carcinoma of the pancreas and papilla of Vater – The prognostic factors influencing the long-term results. A prospective multicentre study. Eur J Surg Oncol 1993;19: 147–161.

2   Rocha Lima CM, Centeno B: Update on pancreatic cancer. Curr Opin Oncol 2002;14:424–430.

3   Wenger FA, Peter F, Zieren J, Steiert A, Jacobi CA, Muller JM: Prognosis factors in carcinoma of the head of the pancreas. Dig Surg 2000;17:29–35.

4   Schafer M, Mullhaupt B, Clavien PA: Evidence-based pancreatic head resection for pancreatic cancer and chronic pancreatitis. Ann Surg 2002;236:137–148.

5   Tsiotos GG, Farnell MB, Sarr MG: Are the results of pancreatectomy for pancreatic cancer improving? World J Surg 1999;23:913–919.

6   Conlon KC, Klimstra DS, Brennan MF: Long-term survival after curative resection for pancreatic ductal adenocarcinoma. Clinicopathologic analysis of 5-year survivors. Ann Surg 1996;223: 273–279.

7   Schima W, Fugger R, Schober E, Oettl C, Wamser P, Grabenwoger F, Ryan JM, Novacek G: Diagnosis and staging of pancreatic cancer: Comparison of mangafodipir trisodium-enhanced MR imaging and contrast-enhanced helical hydro-CT. AJR Am J Roentgenol 2002;179:717–724.

8   Warburg O, Wind F, Neglers E: On the metabolism of tumors in the body; in Warburg O (ed): Metabolism of Tumors. London, Constable, 1930, pp 254–270.

9   Higashi T, Tamaki N, Honda T, Torizuka T, Kimura T, Inokuma T, Ohshio G, Hosotani R, Imamura M, Konishi J: Expression of glucose transporters in human pancreatic tumors compared with increased FDG accumulation in PET study. J Nucl Med 1997;38:1337–1344.

10 Reske SN, Grillenberger KG, Glatting G, Port M, Hildebrandt M, Gansauge F, Beger HG: Overexpression of glucose transporter 1 and increased FDG uptake in pancreatic carcinoma. J Nucl Med 1997;38:1344–1348.

11 Gambhir SS, Czernin J, Schwimmer J, Silverman DH, Coleman RE, Phelps ME: A tabulated summary of the FDG PET literature. J Nucl Med 2001;42(suppl):1S–93S.

12 Klever P, Bares R, Fass J, Büll U, Schumpelick V: PET with fluorine-18 deoxyglucose for pancreatic disease. Lancet 1992;340:1158–1159.

13 Bares R, Klever P, Hellwig D, Hauptmann S, Fass J, Hambuechen U, Zopp L, Mueller B, Buell U, Schumpelick V: Pancreatic cancer detected by positron emission tomography with 18F-labelled deoxyglucose: Method and first results. Nucl Med Commun 1993;14:596–601.

14 Zimny M, Bares R, Fass J, Adam G, Cremerius U, Dohmen B, Klever P, Sabri O, Schumpelick V, Buell U: Fluorine-18 fluorodeoxyglucose positron emission tomography in the differential diagnosis of pancreatic carcinoma: A report of 106 cases. Eur J Nucl Med 1997;24:678–682.

15 Diederichs CG, Staib L, Glatting G, Beger HG, Reske SN: FDG PET: Elevated plasma glucose reduces both uptake and detection rate of pancreatic malignancies. J Nucl Med 1998;39: 1030–1033.

16 Shreve PD: Focal fluorine-18 fluorodeoxyglucose accumulation in inflammatory pancreatic disease. Eur J Nucl Med 1998;25:259–264.

17 Lorenzen J, de Wit M, Buchert R, Igel B, Bohuslavizki KH: Granulation tissue: Pitfall in therapy control with F-18-FDG PET after chemotherapy. Nuklearmedizin 1999;38:333–336.

18 Diederichs CG, Staib L, Glasbrenner B, Guhlmann A, Glatting G, Paul S, Beger HG, Reske SN: F-18 Fluorodeoxyglucose (FDG) and C-reactive protein (CRP). Clin Positron Imaging 1999;2: 131–136.

19 Hamberg LM, Hunter GJ, Alpert NM, Choi NC, Babich JW, Fischman AJ: The dose uptake ratio as an index of glucose metabolism: Useful parameter or oversimplification? J Nucl Med 1994; 35:1308–1312.

20 Hustinx R, Smith RJ, Benard F, Rosenthal DI, Machtay M, Farber LA, Alavi A: Dual time point fluorine-18 fluorodeoxyglucose positron emission tomography: A potential method to differentiate malignancy from inflammation and normal tissue in the head and neck. Eur J Nucl Med 1999; 26:1345–1348.

21 Imdahl A, Nitzsche E, Krautmann F, Hogerle S, Boos S, Einert A, Sontheimer J, Farthmann EH: Evaluation of positron emission tomography with 2-[18F]fluoro-2-deoxy-*D*-glucose for the differentiation of chronic pancreatitis and pancreatic cancer. Br J Surg 1999;86:194–199.

22 Nakamoto Y, Higashi T, Sakahara H, Tamaki N, Kogire M, Doi R, Hosotani R, Imamura M, Konishi J: Delayed (18)F-fluoro-2-deoxy-*D*-glucose positron emission tomography scan for differentiation between malignant and benign lesions in the pancreas. Cancer 2000;89:2547–2554.

23 Nitzsche EU, Hoegerle S, Mix M, Brink I, Otte A, Moser E, Imdahl A: Non-invasive differentiation of pancreatic lesions: Is analysis of FDG kinetics superior to semiquantitative uptake value analysis? Eur J Nucl Med Mol Imaging 2002;29:237–242.

24 Diederichs CG, Staib L, Vogel J, Glasbrenner B, Glatting G, Brambs HJ, Beger HG, Reske SN: Values and limitations of 18F-fluorodeoxyglucose-positron-emission tomography with preoperative evaluation of patients with pancreatic masses. Pancreas 2000;20:109–116.

25 Rose DM, Delbeke D, Beauchamp RD, Chapman WC, Sandler MP, Sharp KW, Richards WO, Wright JK, Frexes ME, Pinson CW, Leach SD: 18Fluorodeoxyglucose-positron emission tomography in the management of patients with suspected pancreatic cancer. Ann Surg 1999;229: 729–737.

26 Sperti C, Pasquali C, Chierichetti F, Liessi G, Ferlin G, Pedrazzoli S: Value of 18-fluorodeoxyglucose positron emission tomography in the management of patients with cystic tumors of the pancreas. Ann Surg 2001;234:675–680.

27 Sendler A, Avril N, Helmberger H, Stollfuss J, Weber W, Bengel F, Schwaiger M, Roder JD, Siewert JR: Preoperative evaluation of pancreatic masses with positron emission tomography using 18F-fluorodeoxyglucose: Diagnostic limitations. World J Surg 2000;24:1121–1129.

28 Fröhlich A, Diederichs CG, Staib L, Vogel J, Beger HG, Reske SN: Detection of liver metastases from pancreatic cancer using FDG PET. J Nucl Med 1999;40:250–255.

29 Nakamoto Y, Higashi T, Sakahara H, Tamaki N, Kogire M, Imamura M, Konishi J: Contribution of PET in the detection of liver metastases from pancreatic tumours. Clin Radiol 1999;54: 248–252.

30 Bares R, Gehl HB, Kaiser HJ, Klever P, Buell U, Guenther R, Schumpelick V: Magnetic resonance imaging (MRI) and positron emission tomography (PET) using fluorine-18 labelled deoxyglucose (FDG) for detection of pancreatic cancer: Comparison and image merging. Eur J Nucl Med 1993; 20:977.

31 Benyounes H, Smith FW, Campbell C, Evans NT, Norton MY, Mikecz P, Heys SD, Bruce D, Eremin O, Sharp PF: Superimposition of PET images using 18F-fluorodeoxyglucose with magnetic resonance images in patients with pancreatic carcinoma. Nucl Med Commun 1995;16: 575–580.

32 Hosten N, Lemke AJ, Wiedenmann B, Bohmig M, Rosewicz S: Combined imaging techniques for pancreatic cancer. Lancet 2000;356:909–910.

33 Beyer T, Townsend DW, Brun T, Kinahan PE, Charron M, Roddy R, Jerin J, Young J, Byars L, Nutt R: A combined PET/CT scanner for clinical oncology. J Nucl Med 2000;41: 1369–1379.

34 Nakata B, Chung YS, Nishimura S, Nishihara T, Sakurai Y, Sawada T, Okamura T, Kawabe J, Ochi H, Sowa M: 18F-fluorodeoxyglucose positron emission tomography and the prognosis of patients with pancreatic adenocarcinoma. Cancer 1997;79:695–699.

35 Zimny M, Fass J, Bares R, Cremerius U, Sabri O, Buechin P, Schumpelick V, Buell U: Fluorodeoxyglucose positron emission tomography and the prognosis of pancreatic carcinoma. Scand J Gastroenterol 2000;35:883–888.

36 Nakata B, Nishimura S, Ishikawa T, Ohira M, Nishino H, Kawabe J, Ochi H, Hirakawa K: Prognostic predictive value of 18F-fluorodeoxyglucose positron emission tomography for patients with pancreatic cancer. Int J Oncol 2001;19:53–58.

37 Maisey NR, Webb A, Flux GD, Padhani A, Cunningham DC, Ott RJ, Norman A: FDG-PET in the prediction of survival of patients with cancer of the pancreas: A pilot study. Br J Cancer 2000;83: 287–293.

38 Higashi T, Sakahara H, Torizuka T, Nakamoto Y, Kanamori S, Hiraoka M, Imamura M, Nishimura Y, Tamaki N, Konishi J: Evaluation of intraoperative radiation therapy for unresectable pancreatic cancer with FDG PET. J Nucl Med 1999;40:1424–1433.

39   Bares R, Klever P, Hauptmann S, Hellwig D, Fass J, Cremerius U, Schumpelick V, Mittermayer C, Büll U: F-18 fluorodeoxyglucose PET in vivo evaluation of pancreatic glucose metabolism for detection of pancreatic cancer. Radiology 1994;192:79–86.

40   Stollfuss JC, Glatting G, Friess H, Kocher F, Berger HG, Reske SN: 2-(Fluorine-18)-fluoro-2-deoxy-*D*-glucose PET in detection of pancreatic cancer: Value of quantitative image interpretation. Radiology 1995;195:339–344.

41   Friess H, Langhans J, Ebert M, Beger HG, Stollfuss J, Reske SN, Buchler MW: Diagnosis of pancreatic cancer by 2[18F]-fluoro-2-deoxy-*D*-glucose positron emission tomography. Gut 1995; 36:771–777.

42   Inokuma T, Tamaki N, Torizuka T, Magata Y, Fujii M, Yonekura Y, Kajiyama T, Ohshio G, Imamura M, Konishi J: Evaluation of pancreatic tumors with positron emission tomography and F-18 fluorodeoxyglucose: Comparison with CT and US. Radiology 1995;195:345–352.

43   Kato T, Fukatsu H, Ito K, Tadokoro M, Ota T, Ikeda M, Isomura T, Ito S, Nishino M, Ishigaki T: Fluorodeoxyglucose positron emission tomography in pancreatic cancer: An unsolved problem. Eur J Nucl Med 1995;22:32–39.

44   Bares R, Dohmen BM, Cremerius U, Fass J, Teusch M, Büll U: Results of positron emission tomography with fluorine-18 labeled fluorodeoxyglucose in differential diagnosis and staging of pancreatic carcinoma. Radiologe 1996;36:435–440.

45   Ho CL, Dehdashti F, Griffeth LK, Buse PE, Balfe DM, Siegel BA: FDG-PET evaluation of indeterminate pancreatic masses. J Comput Assist Tomogr 1996;20:363–369.

46   Keogan MT, Tyler D, Clark L, Branch MS, McDermott VG, DeLong DM, Coleman RE: Diagnosis of pancreatic carcinoma: Role of FDG PET. AJR Am J Roentgenol 1998;171:1565–1570.

47   Rajput A, Stellato TA, Faulhaber PF, Vesselle HJ, Miraldi F: The role of fluorodeoxyglucose and positron emission tomography in the evaluation of pancreatic disease. Surgery 1998;124:793–797.

48   Sendler A, Avril N, Roder JD, Schwaiger M, Siewert JR: Can the extent of pancreatic tumors be evaluated reliably enough by positron emission tomography (PET). Langenbecks Arch Chir Suppl Kongressbd 1998;115:1485–1487.

49   Delbeke D, Rose DM, Chapman WC, Pinson CW, Wright JK, Beauchamp RD, Shyr Y, Leach SD: Optimal interpretation of FDG PET in the diagnosis, staging and management of pancreatic carcinoma. J Nucl Med 1999;40:1784–1791.

50   Koyama K, Okamura T, Kawabe J, Nakata B, Chung KH, Ochi H, Yamada R: Diagnostic usefulness of FDG PET for pancreatic mass lesions. Ann Nucl Med 2001;15:217–224.

51   Papos M, Takacs T, Tron L, Farkas G, Ambrus E, Szakall S Jr, Lonovics J, Csernay L, Pavics L: The possible role of F-18 FDG positron emission tomography in the differential diagnosis of focal pancreatic lesions. Clin Nucl Med 2002;27:197–201.

Michael Zimny, MD
Institute of Nuclear Medicine, Municipal Hospital Hanau
Leimenstrasse 20, DE–63450 Hanau (Germany)
Tel. +49 6181 9551150, Fax +49 6181 9221110, E-Mail zimny@nuklearmedizin-hanau.de

Wiegel T, Höcht S, Sternemann M, Buhr HJ, Hinkelbein W (eds): Controversies in Gastrointestinal
Tumor Therapy. Front Radiat Ther Oncol. Basel, Karger, 2004, vol 38, pp 76–81

....

Adjuvant Radiochemotherapy in Pancreatic Cancer: Contra

Doris Henne-Bruns, Ludger Staib

Department of Visceral and Transplantation Surgery,
University of Ulm, Ulm, Germany

The prognosis of pancreatic cancer still remains poor. This is for several reasons. One reason is the late onset of symptoms, especially in patients with tumors of the pancreatic corpus or tail. Another reason is related to the anatomical location of the pancreas with close relationship to major vessels, like the celiac trunk (hepatic artery, splenic artery), mesenteric artery, and the superior mesenteric vein/portal vein. Because of the close relationship of the pancreas to these vessels, invasion by the tumor can frequently be observed. A further reason for the poor prognosis can be seen in the growth pattern of pancreatic tumors at an early stage with perineural and/or lymphogenous invasion and frequent peritoneal and hematogenous spread.

For the reasons mentioned, not more than 20–30% of patients with pancreatic carcinoma can be resected at the time of diagnosis. In the majority of these patients a pancreatic head carcinoma is found. Only a minor percentage of patients with pancreatic body and tail carcinoma are resectable at the time of diagnosis [1].

In resectable cases, a R0 resection cannot always be achieved, but even for R0-resected patients, the overall 5-year survival rate rarely exceeds more than 25%. Because of this poor prognosis, even in curatively resected patients, extended surgical procedures have been developed in the last 20 years [2]. The extended operations include intra- and retroperitoneal lymphadenectomies as well as in some series portal venous and/or arterial resections.

The idea to improve the prognosis by extended removal of lymphatic tissue was, among others, based on the findings of Ishikawa et al. [2] who in 1988 reported an improvement in the 5-year survival from 9 to 28% for patients who underwent extended intra- and retroperitoneal lymphadenectomy together with

Table 1. Pancreatic carcinoma: results after surgical resection

Author	Number of patients	Median survival months	5-year survival, %
Yeo et al. [4]	81 standard	21	10
	82 radical	20	25
Neoptolemos et al. [5]	440	19.9	
Onoue et al. [6]	69	12	16.1
Kedra et al. [7]	136	18	
Conlon et al. [8]	118	14.3	10.2
Nitecki et al. [9]	186	17.5	6.8
Baumel et al. [10]	555	14	

pancreatic resection. Our own data from Kiel [3] could not reproduce the results published by Ishikawa et al. [2], nor could others (table 1).

Results of Clinical Studies with Extended Lymph Node Dissection

A comparison of the results of different authors is difficult because many parameters vary considerably in the different studies [5, 11–13]. These are for example: (1) the operative technique regarding the extent of lymphadenectomy or the percentage of portal venous resections; (2) the histopathological investigation (number of resected and analyzed lymph nodes); (3) the exact localization of infiltrated tissue, especially at the retroperitoneal resection margin; (4) the differentiation of the tumor; (5) the percentage of ductal adenocarcinomas of the pancreas in the groups of patients analyzed; (6) the distribution of tumor stages in patients with ductal adenocarcinoma within the studies; (7) the percentage of R0-resected patients, and (8) the percentage of patients undergoing adjuvant chemotherapy/radiochemotherapy.

Due to these differences in the published literature it is difficult to judge whether the extend of lymphadenectomy has an impact on the prognosis of patients with adenocarcinoma of the pancreas.

Adjuvant Radiochemotherapy

The intention of adjuvant radiochemotherapy is to avoid or at least postpone local recurrence (radiotherapy) or tumor cell dissemination (chemotherapy).

Table 2. Pancreatic cancer: sites of metastatic spread [14]

	%
Local retroperitoneal recurrence	80
Hepatic metastases	66
peritoneal dissemination	53
Lymph node recurrence	47

Table 3. Pancreatic carcinoma: detection of micrometastases in patients with R0 resections [15–18]

	%
Peritoneal	33–39
Tumor-free lymph nodes	72
Bone marrow	38–69

The rationale behind this is based on autopsy studies as well as on investigations regarding the detection of disseminated tumor cells. Autopsy studies [14] showed that local tumor recurrence or peritoneal or hepatic metastases can frequently be observed, even after curative resections (table 2). Recent data showed, for example, that micrometastatic disease can be detected in peripheral blood samples in patients undergoing curative resections. In lymph nodes, which have conventionally been classified as tumor-free, single tumor cells can be identified in up to 72% and the analysis of peritoneal lavage showed positive results for metastases in about 35% of the patients [15–18] (table 3).

Based on the fact that even after R0 resection local recurrence and distant metastases are frequently observed it seemed to be logical to introduce adjuvant radiochemotherapy into the therapeutic concept of pancreatic carcinoma. Meanwhile, postoperative radiochemotherapy has been performed in several studies.

In 1985 Kalser and Ellenberg [19] published a study in 43 patients with pancreatic carcinoma treated with either surgery alone or postoperative radiochemotherapy. The median survival was 20 months for postoperative radiochemotherapy and 11 months for patients undergoing resection only. Due to the small number of patients this result was not statistically significant. A larger study was published by Yeo et al. [13] in 1997. Their investigation included 173 patients. 99 patients underwent radical resection and a standard protocol with radiochemotherapy postoperatively. 21 patients received intensive postoperative radiotherapy and 53 patients were operated without subsequent adjuvant treatment. The results of this study are shown in table 4. Surprisingly patients receiving the 'intensive' postoperative protocol had a lower median survival than those receiving

Table 4. Postoperative radiochemotherapy (5-FU) after pancreatic resection

Author		Number of patients	Survival months	p
Kalser et al. [19], 1985	OP+RCT	21	20	0.3
	OP	22	11	
Willett et al. [14, 20], 1993	OP+RCT	16	29% 5 years	
	OP	19	18% 5 years	
Yeo et al. [13], 1997	OP+RCTs	99	21	0.002
	OP+RCTi	21	17.5	0.252
	OP	53	13.3	
Klinkenbijl et al. (EORTC) [21], 1999	OP+RCT	60	17.1	0.099
	OP	54	13	
Neoptolemos et al. [22], 2001	OP+RCT	175	15.5	n.s.
	OP	178	16.1	

OP = Surgery; RCT = radiochemotherapy; s = standard protocol; i = intensive protocol.

a standard protocol. Although the authors found a significant difference in the survival time for the group of patients with postoperative adjuvant radiochemotherapy, the benefit of adjuvant therapy is difficult to judge because the published data are a retrospective review of the postoperative treatment and not a prospective randomized trial.

In 1999 Klinkenbijl et al. [21] published the results of a randomized trial on patients with either pancreatic or periampullary cancer who were treated postoperatively with regional radiochemotherapy. The results are shown in table 4. The data showed no statistically significant difference. Although this trial was performed as adjuvant therapy, it has to be mentioned that in about 25% of the observation group and about 20% of the treatment group tumor infiltration of the resection margin has been observed. Therefore, these patients have to be regarded as R1-resected. The largest study regarding adjuvant radiochemotherapy in pancreatic cancer was published by Neoptolemos et al. [22] in 2001. This randomized controlled trial (ESPAC-1) of the European Study Group for Pancreatic Cancer investigated the effect of systemic chemotherapy, radiochemotherapy or both versus observation in a randomized trial by a two-by-two factorial design. The results show that there was no difference in survival between the 175 patients receiving postoperative radiochemotherapy to those without any further adjuvant treatment (n = 178).

Summarizing the results of the published studies it is obvious that to date a significant benefit in survival and quality of life could not be shown for patients with pancreatic cancer treated postoperatively by adjuvant radiochemotherapy. In addition, hospitalization time, toxicity and costs have to be taken into account in relation to the limited life expectancy of less than 20 months after resection. Therefore, to date adjuvant radiochemotherapy in pancreatic cancer cannot be recommended.

References

1   Henne-Bruns D, Vogel I: Does the extent of lymphadenectomy have impact on the prognosis of patients with pancreatic cancer? Onkologie 2002;25:69–71.
2   Ishikawa O, Ohigashi H, Sasaki Y, Kabuto T, Fukuda I, Furukawa H, Imaoka S, Iwanaga T: Practical usefulness of lymphatic and connective tissue clearance for the carcinoma of the pancreatic head. Ann Surg 1988;208:215–220.
3   Henne-Bruns D, Vogel I, Lüttges J, Klöppel G, Kremer B: Surgery for ductal adenocarcinoma of the pancreatic head: Staging, complications and survival after regional versus extended lymphadenectomy. World J Surg 2000;24:595–602.
4   Yeo CJ, Cameron JL, Lillemoe KD, Sohn TA, Campbell KA, Sauter PK, Coleman JA, Abrams RA, Hruban RH: Pancreaticoduodenectomy with or without distal gastrectomy and extended retroperitoneal lymphadenectomy for periampullary adenocarcinoma, part 2. Ann Surg 2002;236:355–368.
5   Neoptolemos JP, Stocken DD, Dunn JA, Almond J, Beger HG, Pederzoli P, Bassi C, Dervenis C, Fernandez-Cruz L, Lacaine F, Buckels J, Deakin M, Adab FA, Sutton R, Imrie C, Ihse I, Tihanyi T, Olah A, Pedrazzoli S, Spooner D, Kerr DJ, Friess H, Büchler MW: Influence of resection margins on survival for patients with pancreatic cancer treated by adjuvant chemoradiation and/or chemotherapy in the ESPAC-1 randomized controlled trial. Ann Surg 2001;234:758–768.
6   Onoue S, Katoh T, Chigira H, Shibata Y, Matsuo K, Suzuki M: Carcinoma of the head of the pancreas. Hepatogastroenterology 2002;49:549–552.
7   Kedra B, Popiela T, Sierzega M, Precht A: Prognostic factors of long-term survival after resective procedures for pancreatic cancer. Hepatogastroenterology 2001;48:1762–1766.
8   Conlon KC, Klimstra DS, Brennan MF: Long-term survival after curative resection for pancreatic ductal adenocarcinoma. Clinicopathologic analysis of 5-year survivors. Ann Surg 1996;223: 273–279.
9   Nitecki SS, Sarr MG, Colby TV: Long-term survival after resection for ductal adenocarcinoma of the pancreas. Is it really improving? Ann Surg 1995;221:59–66.
10 Baumel H, Huguier M, Manderscheid JC: Results of resection for cancer of the exocrine pancreas: A study from the French Association of Surgery. Br J Surg 1994;81:102–107.
11 Pedrazzoli S, Beger HG, Obertop H, Andren-Sandberg A, Fernandez-Del Casillo C, Henne-Bruns D, Lüttgers J, Neoptolemos JP: A surgical and pathological based classification of resective treatment of pancreatic cancer. Dig Surg 1999;16:337–345.
12 Ishikawa O, Ohigashi H, Imaoka S, Furukawa H, Sasaki Y, Fujita M, Kuroda C, Iwanaga T: Preoperative indications for extended pancreatectomy for locally advanced pancreas cancer involving the portal vein. Ann Surg 1992;215:231–236.
13 Yeo CJ, Abrams RA, Grochow LB, Sohn TA, Ord SE, Hruban RH, Zahurak ML, Dooley WC, Coleman JA, Sauer PK, Pitt HA, Lillemoe KD, Cameron JL: Pancreaticoduodenectomy for pancreatic adenocarcinoma: Postoperative adjuvant chemoradiation improves survival. A prospective, single-institution experience. Ann Surg 1997;225(5):621–636.
14 Kayahara M, Nagakawa T, Ueno K, Ohta T, Takeda T, Miyazaki I: An evaluation of radical resection for pancreatic cancer based on the mode of recurrence as determined by autopsy and diagnostic imaging. Cancer 1993;72:2118–2123.
15 Vogel I, Krüger U, Marksen J, Süd E, Kalthoff A, Henne-Bruns D, Kremer B, Juhl H: Disseminated tumor cells in pancreatic cancer. Patients detected by immunocytology: A new prognostic factor. Clin Cancer Res 1999;5:593–599.

16   Gerhard M, Juhl H, Kalthoff H, Schreiber HW, Wagener C, Neumaier M: Specific detection of carcinoembryonic antigen-expressing tumor cells in bone marrow aspirates by polymerase chain reaction. J Clin Oncol 1994;12:725–729.
17   Roder JD, Thorban S, Pantel K, Siegert JR: Micrometastases in bone marrow: Prognostic indicators for pancreatic cancer. World J Surg 1999;23:888–891.
18   Hosch SB, Knöfel WT, Mett S, Stöcklein N, Niendorf A, Brölsch CE, Izbicki JR: Early lymphatic tumor dissemination in pancreatic cancer: Frequency and prognostic significance. Pancreas 1997; 15:154–159.
19   Kalser MH, Ellenberg SS: Pancreatic Cancer. Adjuvant combined radiation and chemotherapy following curative resection. Arch Surg 1985;120:899–903.
20   Willett CG, Lewandrowski K, Warshaw AL, Efird J, Compton CC: Resection margins in carcinoma of the head of the pancreas. Implications for radiation therapy. Ann Surg 1993;217:144–148.
21   Klinkenbijl JH, Jeekel J, Sahmoud T, van Pel R, Couvreur ML, Veenhof CH, Arnaud JP, Gonzalez DG, de Wit LT, Hennipman A, Wils J: Adjuvant radiotherapy and 5-fluorouracil after curative resection of cancer of the pancreas and periampullary region. Phase III trial of the EORTC Gastrointestinal Tract Cancer Cooperative Group. Ann Surg 1999;230:776–784.
22   Neoptolemos JP, Dunn JA, Stocken DD, Almond J, Link K, Beger H, Bassi C, Falconi M, Pederzoli P, Dervenis C, Fernandez-Cruz L, Lacaine F, Pap A, Spooner D, Kerr DJ, Friess H, Büchler MW: Adjuvant chemoradiotherapy and chemotherapy in resectable pancreatic cancer: A randomised controlled trial. Lancet 2001;358:1576–1585.

Prof. Dr. Doris Henne-Bruns
Department of Visceral and Transplantation Surgery
University of Ulm, DE–89070 Ulm (Germany)
Tel. +49 731 500 27200, Fax +49 731 500 27209
E-Mail doris.henne-bruns@medizin.uni-ulm.de

Wiegel T, Höcht S, Sternemann M, Buhr HJ, Hinkelbein W (eds): Controversies in Gastrointestinal
Tumor Therapy. Front Radiat Ther Oncol. Basel, Karger, 2004, vol 38, pp 82–86

....
Adjuvant Radiochemotherapy for Pancreatic Cancer – Why We Might Need It Even More

J. Fleckenstein, C. Rübe

Department of Radiotherapy, Saarland University Medical School,
Homburg, Germany

There is a lasting controversy about the value of adjuvant therapy in resected pancreatic cancer. Does the indication depend solely on the resection margin status? Is radiochemotherapy indicated or rather chemotherapy alone? Is there any indication at all?

We claim that adjuvant radiochemotherapy seems to be the most promising type of adjuvant treatment in pancreatic cancer.

At first glance the recent results of the ESPAC-1 and ESPAC-1(R1) trial give little support for this assumption. In 2001 Neoptolemos et al. [1, 2] reported the results of this randomized controlled trial that was designed to assess the role of adjuvant radiochemotherapy and chemotherapy in pancreatic cancer. 541 patients were eligible and had had potentially curative surgery before. Clinicians of 61 cancer centers could select between three randomization options: a two-by-two factorial design (radiochemotherapy vs. chemotherapy vs. both radiochemotherapy and chemotherapy vs. no adjuvant therapy), which was used in 285 patients, or (finally in 68 patients) radiochemotherapy only (radiochemotherapy vs. no adjuvant therapy), or (in 188 patients) chemotherapy only (chemotherapy vs. no adjuvant therapy) which included the possibility of 'background radiochemotherapy'. This shows that the trial actually consisted of three parallel studies. Nevertheless an 'overall' conclusion was drawn. The overall results showed no benefit for adjuvant radiochemotherapy (median survival 15.5 months with radiochemotherapy vs. 16.1 months without) while there was evidence of a survival benefit for adjuvant chemotherapy (median survival 19.7 months with chemotherapy vs. 14.0 months without; p = 0.0005).

Resection margin status was found to be an influential prognostic factor. 19% of the 541 patients had R1 resection. Their median survival was 10.9 vs. 16.9 months survival for patients with R0 margins. In this subgroup analysis of patients with R1 resection no survival difference between radiochemotherapy and chemotherapy was found. The authors concluded that because of the revealed benefit of adjuvant chemotherapy, regardless of the resection status, this track should be followed in the future by means of further randomized trials [1, 2].

As Abrams et al. [3] pointed out in the commentary of this trial, the 'pooling' of the results of the 3 studies led to problematic classifications, e.g. almost one third of the 'no chemotherapy' patients received chemoradiation, as did a similar portion of 'chemotherapy' patients. In addition to that, the administered irradiation dose was not uniform (40 Gy were prescribed, which can be considered as a low dose anyway, but it was left to the radiation oncologist to give up to 60 Gy) and information about radiotherapeutic quality assurance was lacking [3].

After all this trial has to be considered as underpowered to answer the question about the best adjuvant treatment.

Considering other phase-III trials, the first one was conducted by the Gastrointestinal Study Group (GITSG) starting in the mid 1970s. Patients either received no adjuvant therapy or adjuvant split-course radiochemotherapy (40 Gy in 6 weeks with a mid 2-week break, 2 cycles of 5-FU simultaneously) followed by maintenance 5-FU. Patient accrual was poor, only 43 patients were randomized. Those who received radiochemotherapy showed a median survival of 21 months, a 2-year survival of 43% and a 5-year survival of 19% which was significantly different from the control group (11 months, 18 and 5%, respectively) [4]. These results were confirmed in an additional non-randomized patient cohort (n = 30) treated with the same radiochemotherapeutic modality [5].

The results of the two GITSG trials are still not convincing especially due to the small sample sizes, slow patient accrual rates, and the lack of a control group in the follow-up study. Nevertheless the data had to be considered as encouraging.

Based on the standard regimen of the GITSG trials, Yeo et al. [6] confirmed their results in a single-institution trial. 173 patients with pancreatic cancer in the head or uncinate process, in whom pancreaticoduodenectomy had been performed, could select between three treatment options: (1) standard therapy (elected by 99 patients) consisting of radiotherapy to the pancreatic bed (40–45 Gy) given with two 3-day 5-FU courses and followed by weekly bolus 5-FU for 4 months (same regimen as in the GITSG-trials); (2) intensive therapy (21 patients) consisting of radiotherapy to the pancreatic bed (50.4–57.6 Gy) with prophylactic hepatic irradiation (23.4–27 Gy) given with and followed by infusional 5-FU plus leucovorin for 5 of 7 days for 4 months, or (3) no therapy (53 patients). The authors found that the use of postoperative adjuvant radio-chemotherapy was a predictor of improved survival (median survival 19.5 months compared to 13.5 months without therapy; p = 0.003). The intensive therapy group had no survival advantage when compared to that of the standard therapy group. Other most powerful predictors of outcome were tumor diameter (<3 cm), intraoperative blood loss and status of resection margins [6].

The European Organization for Research and Treatment of Cancer (EORTC) completed a phase-III trial comparing split-course radiochemotherapy as used in the GITSG trial (without maintenance chemotherapy) to observation. Included were 218 patients with pancreatic head (55% of all patients) or periampullary cancer (45%) and histologically proven adenocarcinoma who were randomized after resection. The median duration of survival was 24.5 months for the treatment group and 19.0 months for the observation group (p = 0.208). When stratifying for tumor location the differences were still not significant. The adjuvant radiochemotherapy was safe and well tolerated. The authors concluded that the routine use of adjuvant radiochemotherapy is not warranted as standard treatment in cancer of the head of the pancreas or periampullary region [7].

This interpretation of the results should be viewed tentatively because patients with positive margins have been included without stratification due to the lack of radiation therapy quality assurance and the lack of maintenance therapy in the adjuvant regimen.

Admitting that, when considering historical and more recent clinical trials (randomized as well as non-randomized), there is no overwhelming evidence for adjuvant radiochemotherapy in pancreatic cancer, one still has to cope with the extremely disappointing results of surgery alone. Assuming that about 15% of all patients with pancreatic cancer can undergo potentially curative resection, their 5-year survival rate is less than 20% [8, 9]. Focusing on the subgroup of patients with favorable prognostic parameters (R0 resection, small tumor diameter, no positive lymph nodes), the 5-year survival rate is still no more than 36% [9–12].

Our strong opinion is that there is still a lot of room for further sustained improvement in therapy outcome and that adjuvant radiochemotherapy will play an important role in this setting. This hope about the future can be derived from strong improvements in each single treatment modality. There been a strong decrease in the morbidity and mortality of pancreatoduodenectomy over the past 20 years [13, 14]. Meanwhile 5-FU sequencing and administration have been advanced and gemcitabine has not only shown significant radiosensitizing properties, but has also been approved for use against pancreatic cancer.

Besides that the remarkable progress in radiation therapy planning and radiation biology allowed continuous escalation of treatment dose and optimization of treatment schemes.

From a modern radiobiological point of view a radiotherapeutic split course technique, such as used as 'standard therapy' in the GITSG trial, seems obsolete because of the presumably fast recovery of tumor cells. A total irradiation dose of 40 Gy seems too small with regard to lasting tumor control. Instead of that cumulative doses of at least 45 Gy (up to 55 Gy in a small ('boost') volume) may be prescribed.

In this context the possibility of additional intraoperative radiotherapy (IORT), which, as matter of fact, is not available in many centers, has to be mentioned. Using IORT in combination with radiochemotherapy in the adjuvant setting might at least enhance freedom of local failure. Whilst in unresectable adenocarcinoma of the pancreas IORT at least proved to be highly effective due to pain alleviation, in the adjuvant situation no clear indication can be derived from the already existing data. There seems to be a tendency to improved local tumor control and median survival time if IORT is used in combination with external beam radiation therapy following curative resection [15, 16].

These treatment possibilities are not or, at most, partially included in the above-mentioned studies.

In a recent publication of a pilot study, Wilkowski et al. [17] presented a treatment scheme using concomitant and sequential gemcitabine and cisplatin with radiotherapy (50 Gy) in 57 patients with pancreatic cancer. 19 of these patients had resection before (R1 and/or pN+), 33 patients had unresectable tumors and 5 had local recurrent disease. The treatment scheme was feasible, the side effects were justifiable. No gastrointestinal toxicities of grade III or IV were observed. Hematologic toxicities were of only minor clinical relevance (1 neutropenic infection, 1 thrombopenic epistasis). The median survival time of the postoperative patients was 15.1 months [17].

In a 1998 editorial review Regine and Abrams [18] updated the status of adjuvant therapy for pancreatic cancer and introduced the RTOG 97-04 phase-III trial that incorporates more recently gained knowledge in this context. In the adjuvant setting pre- and post-chemoradiation 5-FU vs. pre- and post-chemoradiation gemcitabine were prospectively randomized. In both arms radiotherapy consists of 50.4 at 1.8 Gy/fraction (field reduction at 45 Gy) and 5-FU (250 mg/m^2/day) as continuous infusion is given simultaneously [18]. Unfortunately there is no treatment arm consisting of chemotherapy alone to compare differences in local failure and survival. Still we expect this well-designed trial (the results have not been published yet) to be important in clarifying the role of adjuvant radiochemotherapy in pancreatic cancer.

We conclude that in this setting 'state of the art' radiochemotherapy seems far too effective and potentially beneficial to be omitted in future clinical trials.

References

1   Neoptolemos JP, Dunn JA, Stocken DD, et al: Adjuvant chemoradiotherapy and chemotherapy in resectable pancreatic cancer: A randomised controlled trial. Lancet 2001;358:1576–1585.
2   Neoptolemos JP, Stocken DD, Dunn JA, et al: Influence of resection margins on survival for patients with pancreatic cancer treated by adjuvant chemoradiation and/or chemotherapy in the ESPAC-1 randomised controlled trial. Ann Surg 2001;234:758–768.
3   Abrams RA, Lillemoe KD, Piantadosi S: Continuing controversy over adjuvant therapy of pancreatic cancer. Lancet 2001;358:1565–1566.
4   Kalser MH, Ellenberg SS: Pancreatic cancer. Adjuvant combined radiation and chemotherapy following curative resection. Arch Surg 1985;120:899–903.
5   Gastrointestinal Tumor Study Group: Further evidence of effective adjuvant combined radiation and chemotherapy following curative resection of pancreatic cancer. Cancer 1987;59:2006–2010.
6   Yeo CJ, Abrams RA, Grochow LB, et al: Pancreaticoduodenectomy for pancreatic adenocarcinoma: Postoperative adjuvant chemoradiation improves survival. A prospective, single institution experience. Ann Surg 1997;225:621–636.
7   Klinkenbijl JH, Jeekel J, Sahmoud T, et al: Adjuvant radiotherapy and 5-fluorouracil after curative resection of cancer of the pancreas and periampullary region. Phase III trial of the EORTC Gastrointestinal Tract Cancer Cooperative Group. Ann Surg 1999;230:776–784.
8   Douglass H: Adjuvant therapy for pancreatic cancer. World J Surg 1995;19:170–174.
9   Nitecki SS, Sarr MG, Colby TV, et al: Long-term survival after resection for ductal adenocarcinoma of the pancreas. Is it really improving? Ann Surg 1995;221:59–66.
10 Geer RJ, Brennan MF: Prognostic indicators for survival after resection of pancreatic adenocarcinoma. Am J Surg 1993;165:68–73.
11 Gudjonsson B: Cancer of the pancreas: 50 years of surgery. Cancer 1987;60:2284–2303.
12 Piorkowski RJ, Believernicht SW, Lawrence W, et al: Pancreatic and periampullary carcinoma: Experience with 200 patients over a 12-year period. Am J Surg 1982;143:189–193.
13 Yeo CJ, Cameron JL, Lillemoe KD, et al: Pancreaticoduodenectomy for cancer of the head of the pancreas. Two hundred and on patients. Ann Surg 1995;221:721–733.
14 Yeo CJ, Cameron JL, Sohn TA, et al: 650 consecutive pancreaticoduodenectomies in the 1990s: Pathology, complications, outcomes. Ann Surg 1997;226:248–260.
15 Willich N, Krämling H-J, Rübe C: Study on IORT in 44 patients with unresectable adenocarcinoma of the pancreas; in Schildberg FW (ed): Intraoperative Radiation Therapy. Proc 4th Int Symp, Munich, 1993, pp 311–323.
16 Kokubo M, Nishimura Y, Shibamoto Y, et al: Analysis of the clinical benefit of intraoperative radiotherapy in patients undergoing macroscopically curative resection for pancreatic cancer. Int J Radiat Oncol Biol Phys 2000;48:1081–1087.
17 Wilkowski R, Thoma M, Heinemann V, et al: Radiochemotherapy with gemcitabine and cisplatin in pancreatic cancer – Feasible and effective (in German). Strahlenther Onkol 2003;179:78–86.
18 Regine WF, Abrams RA: Adjuvant therapy for pancreatic cancer: Back to the future. Int J Radiat Oncol Biol Phys 1998;42:59–63.

Dr. Jochen Fleckenstein
Department of Radiotherapy, Saarland University Medical School
DE–66421 Homburg/Saar (Germany)
Tel. +49 684 1162 4838, Fax +49 684 1162 4819, E-Mail rajfle@uniklinik-saarland.de

Wiegel T, Höcht S, Sternemann M, Buhr HJ, Hinkelbein W (eds): Controversies in Gastrointestinal
Tumor Therapy. Front Radiat Ther Oncol. Basel, Karger, 2004, vol 38, pp 87–93

....

Radiochemotherapy in Unresectable Pancreatic Cancer

Stefan Höcht, Thomas Wiegel, Alessandra Siegmann,
Wolfgang Hinkelbein

Clinic for Radiation Oncology and Radiotherapy,
Charité, Campus Benjamin Franklin, Berlin, Germany

In Western countries, cancer of the exocrine pancreas is one of the major causes of cancer-related mortality and morbidity. With an incidence of roughly 1:10,000, pancreatic cancer is among the six most common malignant diseases. In untreated patients, median survival is only 4–6 months [1]. Somewhat depending on the site of the organ involved, locally progressive disease causes pain, jaundice, gastric outlet stenosis, nonspecific upper abdominal symptoms or simply a loss of body mass. Detection at an early stage of the disease is a rare event. Although considerable success has been made in recent years in diagnostic procedures, disseminated disease, especially peritoneal seeding, can often only be ruled out by laparoscopy or laparotomy [2, 3].

Complete operative removal of all malignant tissue is the only way to cure pancreatic cancer, resulting in 5-year-survival rates in the range of 2–25% [4–6]. Adjuvant therapy after curative resection is still under debate with different attitudes across the Atlantic Ocean. While postoperative or preoperative radiochemotherapy is an established standard of care in the United States of America [7], this is not the case in Western Europe. Due to the lack of statistical power, impeding imbalances by trial design, inclusion criteria, outdated radiotherapy techniques or split course radiotherapy treatment, etc., a variety of conflicting phase-III studies with inconclusive results leaves the main questions unanswered but offers room for extensive debates [8–12].

In metastatic disease, chemotherapy with gemcitabine as single agent therapy is well tolerated and has replaced 5-fluorouracil since it was shown to improve quality of life in terms of a so-called 'clinical benefit response', and hence is nowadays regarded as standard [13, 14].

Chemoradiation as Standard of Good Clinical Practice in Locally Advanced Non-Metastatic Disease

A substantial proportion of patients presents with neither resectable nor metastatic but locally advanced disease, and in these patients radiochemotherapy is able to offer an estimated gain of about 3–6 months in median survival. Starting in the late 1960s a growing body of evidence has evolved from small phase-II and phase-III trials showing median survival rates in the order of 8–14 months for patients treated that way (table 1) [15–29].

Still not every patient with locally advanced non-metastatic disease is an ideal candidate for radiochemotherapy. Sometimes severe side effects of therapy have to be balanced against the potential benefits. Most authors agree on certain selection criteria for offering chemoradiation: there should be no weight loss of more than 10–15%; patients should be in good to fair general condition with a Karnofsky index of at least 60%; less than 70 years of age, and have adequate hepatic, renal and bone marrow functions. To be honest, one has to admit that these criteria per se define a subpopulation with a better prognosis than average, making it even more difficult to define the real benefits of this therapy as reliable data comparing state-of-the-art chemoradiation, chemotherapy and best supportive care merely do not exist.

Patients with locally advanced unresectable pancreatic cancer generally do have symptoms of their disease, making the definition of side effects of therapy a difficult topic to assess. Besides hematologic toxicity, which can easily be attributed to chemotherapy and radiation, nausea and vomiting, fatigue, mucositis and diarrhea are complaints of up to 75 (grade II) and 10–35% (grade III) of the patients treated. In some of the articles, high rates of stent complications, cholangitis and hepatitis are mentioned as well. Defining the real benefits of therapy would therefore mandate utilization of tools such as a quality-of-life-adjusted survival analysis (Q-TWiST) [30]. Decreasing side effects and shortening overall treatment time should definitely be aims of further research on modifications of therapy [26]. Still long-lasting palliation of symptoms, such as severe pain, is often achieved by radiochemotherapy, and the development of very potent anti-emetics and hemopoietic growth factors within the last decade has made supportive care easier thus increasing the achievable therapeutic gain.

On the other hand, there is a proportion of patients who become operable after definitive (in that case neoadjuvant) radiochemotherapy, leading quite in the opposite direction: Aiming to increase the response rates of preoperative chemoradiation one will very likely have to accept an increase in toxic side effects of therapy as well. Combining standard-fractionated radiotherapy to 45–54 Gy with continuous infusion 5-fluorouracil as radiosensitizer has evolved to a widely accepted standard of care even though in pancreatic cancer

Table 1. Results of definitive radiochemotherapy in pancreatic cancer

Reference	Patients n	RT dose Gy	CTX[1]	Median survival months
Moertel et al. [15], 1969	32	35–40	–	6
	32	35–40	5-FU	10
Moertel et al. [16], 1981	86	60 (10 weeks)	5-FU	9
	83	40	5-FU	12
	25	60 (10 weeks)	–	6
GITSG [17], 1985	70	40	ADM	8
	73	60 (10 weeks)	5-FU	8
Klaassen et al. [18], 1985	44	–	5-FU	8
	47	40	5-FU+5FU mt	8
GITSG [19], 1988	21	40	5-FU+SMF	8
	22	–	SMF	11
Seydel et al. [20], 1990	18	54	5-FU+SMF mt	8
Treurniet-Donker et al. [21], 1990	40	50	5-FU	9
Boz et al. [22], 1991	22	45–54	5-FU	8
Picus et al. [23], 1994	34	60	5-FU	8
Moertel et al. [24], 1994	22	45–54	5-FU	13
Wagener et al. [25], 1996	53	40	5-FU+CE	11
Prott et al. [26], 1997	32	45	5-FU	13
Nguyen et al. [27], 1997	23	60	DDP	10
Terk et al. [28], 1997	55	54	SPF	17
Kornek et al. [29], 2000	38	55	5-FU/LV/DDP	14
Crane et al. [34], 2002	48	30	GEM	10
	60	30	5-FU	9

[1]Chemotherapy substances: ADM = Adriamycin; CE = cis-platinum, epirubicin; DDP = cis-platinum; 5-FU = 5-fluorouracil; GEM = gemcitabine; LV = leucovorin; SMF = streptozotocin, mitomycin C, 5-fluorouracil; SPF = streptozotocin, cis-platinum, 5-fluorouracil; mt = maintenance therapy.

there is less evidence for the superiority of continuous infusion application than in adjuvant treatment of rectal cancer [31–33].

Probably depending more on the definition of the terms 'marginally resectable' and 'unresectable' than on the actual protocol of therapy chosen, some 20% of locally advanced non-metastatic pancreatic cancer patients become resectable after neoadjuvant chemoradiation, and up to 20% of all patients develop metastatic disease while under neoadjuvant treatment [29, 32, 34–36]. Under evaluation are chemoradiation protocols with multiple chemo-therapeutic agents such as 5-fluorouracil, leucovorin, cis-platinum, mitomycin C, taxanes and gemcitabine in various combinations, and single agent regimes with taxanes and gemcitabine [29, 34, 37–40].

Perspectives

Special interest is focusing on gemcitabine, as it is known to be a potent radiosensitizer and is well tolerated as single-agent standard therapy in metastatic disease. Obviously gemcitabine potentiates not only radiation effects on tumors but on surrounding normal tissues as well. Critical factors are the timing between the administration of chemotherapy and radiotherapy, tolerable dosage, infusion rate and frequency, especially in combination with 5-fluorouracil, and the radiotherapy volume needed [34, 41–44]. In general, maximum tolerable doses of gemcitabine in combination with radiotherapy are in the range of 200–350 mg/m^2/week if not given directly simultaneously but separated from radiation by several hours to up to 2 days; whereas combination protocols with 5-fluorouracil describe dose-limiting toxicities at levels as low as 50 mg/m^2/week. Given the existing but still modest systemic activity of gemcitabine in disseminated disease, the obvious need for dose reduction of gemcitabine in combination therapy makes short-term hypofractionated radiotherapy an attractive schedule as it would not withhold systemically active levels of the drug for a longer time period and still allow a high radiation dose intensity [34, 45].

Aside from clinical trials, a conservative approach in the management of patients with locally advanced pancreatic cancer with standard fractionation and doses of radiation and 5-fluorouracil as continuous infusion should be recommended. The need for properly designed, large multicenter phase-III trials cannot be overestimated.

References

1   Niederhuber J, Brennan M, Menck H: The national cancer data base report on pancreatic cancer. Cancer 1995;76:1671–1677.
2   Hochwald S, Rofsky N, Dobryansky M, Shamamian P, Marcus S: Magnetic resonance imaging with magnetic resonance cholangiopancreatography accurately predicts resectability of pancreatic carcinoma. J Gastrointest Surg 1999;3:506–511.
3   Merchant N, Conlon K, Saigo P, Dougherty E, Brennan M: Positive peritoneal cytology predicts unresectability of pancreatic adenocarcinoma. J Am Coll Surg 1999;188:421–426.
4   Bramhall S, Allum W, Jones A, Allwood A, Cummins C, Neoptolemos J: Treatment and survival in 13,560 patients with pancreatic cancer, and incidence of the disease, in the West Midlands: An epidemiological study. Br J Surg 1995;82:111–115.
5   Conlon K, Klimstra D, Brennan M: Long-term survival after curative resection for pancreatic ductal adenocarcinoma. Clinicopathologic analysis of 5-year survivors. Ann Surg 1996;223:273–279.
6   Birkmeyer J, Warshaw A, Finlayson S, Grove M, Tosteson A: Relationship between hospital volume and late survival after pancreaticoduodenectomy. Surgery 1999;126:178–183.
7   Abbruzzese J: Postoperative and preoperative adjuvant therapy for pancreatic cancer: Controversy and promise; in American Society of Clinical Oncology (eds): 2001 Educational Book. Baltimore, Lippincott Williams & Wilkins, 2001, pp 72–76.
8   Gastrointestinal Tumor Study Group: Further evidence of effective adjuvant combined radiation and chemotherapy following curative resection of pancreatic cancer. Cancer 1987;59:2006–2010.

9   Neoptolemos J, Dunn J, Stocken D, Almond J, Link K, Beger H, Bassi C, Falconi M, Pederzoli P, Dervenis C, Fernandez-Cruz L, Lacaine F, Pap A, Spooner D, Kerr D, Friess H, Büchler M, for the ESPAC: Adjuvant chemoradiotherapy in resectable pancreatic cancer: A randomized controlled trial. Lancet 2001;358:1576–1585.

10 Klinkenbijl JH, Jeekel J, Sahmoud T, van Pel R, Couvreur ML, Veenhof CH, Arnaud JP, Gonzalez DG, de Wit LT, Hennipman A, Wils J: Adjuvant radiotherapy and 5-fluoro-uracil after curative resection of cancer of the pancreas and periampullary region: phase III trial of the EORTC gastrointestinal tract cancer cooperative group. Ann Surg 1999;230:776–782.

11 Wiegel T, Runkel N, Frommhold H, Rübe C, Hinkelbein W: Strahlentherapeutische Strategien in der multimodalen Therapie des resektablen und nicht resektablen Pankreaskarzinoms. Strahlenther Onkol 2000;176:299–306.

12 Terwee C, Nieven van Dijkum E, Gouma D, Bakkevold K, Klinkenbijl J, Wade T, van Wagensveld B, Wong A, van der Meulen J: Pooling of prognostic studies in cancer of the pancreatic head and periampullary region: The triple P study. Tripple P study group. Eur J Surg 2000;166:706–712.

13 Burris H, Moore M, Andersen J, Green M, Rothenberg M, Modiano M, Cripps M, Portenoy R, Storniolo A, Tarassoff P, Nelson R, Dorr F, Stephens C, Von Hoff D: Improvements in survival and clinical benefit with gemcitabine as first-line therapy for patients with advanced pancreas cancer. J Clin Oncol 1997;15:2403–2413.

14 Rothenberg M, Moore M, Cripps M, Andersen J, Portenoy R, Burris H, Green M, Tarassoff P, Brown T, Casper E, Storniolo A, Von Hoff D: A phase II trial of gemcitabine in patients with 5-FU refractory pancreas cancer. Ann Oncol 1996;7:347–353.

15 Moertel C, Childs D, Reitermeier R, Colby M, Holbrook M: Combined 5-fluorouracil and supervoltage radiation therapy for locally unresectable gastrointestinal cancer. Lancet 1969;ii: 865–867.

16 Moertel C, Frytak S, Hahn R, O'Connell M, Reitemeier R, Rubin J, Schutt A, Weiland L, Childs D, Holbrook M, Lavin P, Livstone E, Spiro H, Knowlton A, Kalser M, Barkin J, Lessner H, Mann-Kaplan R, Ramming K, Douglas H, Thomas P. Nave H, Bateman J, Lokich J, Brooks J, Chaffey J, Corson J, Zamcheck M, Novak J: Therapy for locally unresectable pancreatic carcinoma: A randomized comparison of high dose (6000 rads) radiation alone, moderate dose radiation (4000 rads + 5-fluorouracil) and high dose radiation and fluorouracil. Cancer 1981;48: 1705–1710.

17 Gastrointestinal Tumor Study Group: Radiation therapy combined with adriamycin or 5-fluorouracil for the treatment of locally unresectable pancreatic cancer. Cancer 1985;56:2563–2568.

18 Klaassen D, MacIntyre J, Catton G: Treatment of locally unresectable cancer of the stomach and pancreas: A randomized comparison of 5-fluorouracil alone with radiation plus concurrent and maintenance 5-fluorouracil. J Clin Oncol 1985:3:373–378.

19 Gastrointestinal Tumor Study Group: Treatment of locally unresectable carcinoma of the pancreas: Comparison of combined modality therapy (chemotherapy plus radiotherapy) to chemotherapy alone. J Natl Cancer Inst 1988;80:751–755.

20 Seydel H, Stablein D, Leichman, Kinzie J, Thomas P: Hyperfractionated radiation and chemotherapy for unresectable localized adenocarcinoma of the pancreas. Cancer 1990;65:1478–1482.

21 Treurniet-Donker A, van Mierlo M, van Putten W: Localized unresectable pancreatic cancer. Int J Radiat Oncol Biol Phys 1990;18:59–62.

22 Boz G, Paoli A, Roncadin M, Franchin G, Galligioni E, Arcicasa M, Bortolus R, Gobitti C, Minatel E, Innocente R: Radiation therapy combined with chemotherapy for inoperable pancreatic carcinoma. Tumori 1991;77:61–64.

23 Picus J, Dickerson G, Logie K: A phase II study of unresectable pancreatic cancer treated with 5-FU and leucovorin with radiation therapy. Proc Am Soc Clin Oncol 1994;13:A208.

24 Moertel C, Gunderson L, Mailliard J, McKenna P, Martenson J, Burch P, Cha S: Early evaluation of combined fluorouracil and leucovorin as radiation enhancer for locally unresectable, residual or recurrent gastrointestinal carcinoma. J Clin Oncol 1994;12:21–27.

25 Wagener D, Hoogenraad W, Rougier P, Lusinchi A, Taal B, Veenhof C, de Graeff A, Conroy T, Curran D, Sahmoud T, Wils J: Results of a phase II trial of epirubicin and cisplatin (EP) before and after irradiation and 5-fluorouracil in locally advanced pancreatic cancer: An EORTC GITCCG study. Eur J Cancer 1996;32:1310–1313.

26 Prott F, Schönekäs K, Preusser P, Ostkamp K, Wagner W, Micke O, Pötter R, Sulkowski U, Rübe C, Berns T, Willich N: Combined treatment with accelerated radiotherapy and chemotherapy in patients with locally advanced inoperable carcinoma of the pancreas. Br J Cancer 1997;75:597–601.

27 Nguyen T, Theobald S, Rougier P, Ducreux M, Lusinchi A, Bardet E, Eymard J-C, Conroy T, Francois E, Seitz J-F, Perrier H, Bugat R, Ychou M: Multicentric pilot study of simultaneous high dose external irradiation and daily cisplatin in unresectable, non-metastatic adenocarcinoma of the pancreas. Proc Am Soc Clin Oncol 1997;16:A299.

28 Terk M, Turhal N, Mandeli J, Kocheril P, Lavagnini P, Dalton J, Snady H, Cooperman A, Bruckner H: Long term follow-up of combined modality therapy for unresectable pancreatic cancer. Proc Am Soc Clin Oncol 1997:16:A307.

29 Kornek G, Schratter-Sehn A, Marczell A, Depisch D, Karner J, Krauss G, Haider K, Kwasny W, Locker G, Scheithauer W: Treatment of unresectable, locally advanced pancreatic adenocarcinoma with combined radiochemotherapy with 5-fluorouracil, leucovorin and cisplatin. Br J Cancer 2000;82:98–103.

30 Glasziou P, Cole B, Gelber R, Hilden J, Simes R: Quality adjusted survival analysis with repeated quality of life measures. Stat Med 1998;17:1215–1229.

31 Poen J, Collins H, Niederhuber J, Oberhelman H, Vierra M, Bastidas A, Young H, Slosberg E, Jeffrey B, Longacre T, Fisher G, Goffinet D: Chemo-radiotherapy for localized pancreatic cancer: Increased dose intensity and reduced acute toxicity with concomitant radiotherapy and protracted venous infusion 5-fluorouracil. Int J Radiat Oncol Biol Phys 1998;40:93–99.

32 Mehta V, Poen J, Ford J Oberhelman H, Vierra M, Bastidas A, Fisher G: Protracted venous infusion 5-fluorouracil with concomitant radiotherapy compared with bolus 5-fluorouracil for unresectable pancreatic cancer. Am J Clin Oncol 2001;24:155–159.

33 O'Connell M, Martenson J, Wieand H, Krook J, Macdonald J, Haller D, Mayer R, Gunderson L, Rich T: Improving adjuvant therapy for rectal cancer by combining protracted-infusion fluorouracil with radiation therapy after curative surgery. N Engl J Med 1994;331:502–507.

34 Crane C, Abbruzzese J, Evans D, Wolff R, Ballo M, Delclos M, Milas L, Mason K, Charnsangavej C, Pisters P, Lee j, Lenzi R, Vauthey J, Wong A, Phan T, Nguyen Q, Janjan N: Is the therapeutic index better with gemcitabine based chemoradiation than with 5-fluorouracil-based chemoradiation in locally advanced pancreatic cancer? Int J Radiat Oncol Biol Phys 2002;52:1293–1302.

35 White R, Hurwitz H, Morse M, Lee C, Anscher M, Paulson E, Gottfried M, Baillie J, Branch M, Jowell P, McGrath K, Clary B, Pappas T, Tyler D: Neoadjuvant chemoradiation for localized adenocarcinoma of the pancreas. Ann Surg Oncol 2001;8:758–765.

36 Foo M, Gunderson L, Nagorney D, McIlrath D, Van Heerden J, Robinow J, Kvols L, Martenson J, Cha S: Patterns of failure in grossly resected pancreatic ductal adenocarcinoma treated with adjuvant irradiation ± 5-fluorouracil. Int J Radiat Oncol Biol Phys 1993;26:483–489.

37 Pisters PW, Wolff RA, Janjan NA, Cleary KR, Charnsangavej C, Crane CN, Lenzi R, Vauthey JN, Lee JE, Abbruzzese JL, Evans DB: Preoperative paclitaxel and concurrent rapid-fractionation radiation for resectable pancreatic adenocarcinoma: Toxicities, histologic response rates, and event-free outcome. J Clin Oncol 2002;20:2537–2544.

38 Rau, H, Wichmann M, Wilkowski R, Heinemann V, Sackmann M, Helmberger T, Dühmke E, Schildberg F: Chirurgische Therapie des lokal fortgeschrittenen und primär inoperablen Pankreaskarzinoms nach neoadjuvanter präoperativer Radiochemotherapie. Chirurg 2002;73:132–137.

39 Ikeda M, Okada S, Tokuuye K, Ueno H, Okusaka T: A phase I trial of weekly gemcitabine and concurrent radiotherapy in patients with locally advanced pancreatic cancer. Br J Cancer 2002;86:1551–1554.

40 Safran H, Moore T, Iannitti D, Dipetrillo T, Akerman P, Cioffi W, Harrington D, Quirk D, Rathore R, Cruff D, Vakharia J, Vora S, Savarese D, Wanebo H: Paclitaxel and concurrent radiation for locally advanced pancreatic cancer. Int J Radiat Oncol Biol Phys 2001;49:1275–1279.

41 Storniolo A, Enas N, Brown C, Voi M, Rothenberg M, Schilsky R: An investigational new drug treatment program for patients with gemcitabine: Results for over 3000 patients with pancreatic carcinoma. Cancer 1999;85:1261–1268.

42 Van Putten J, Groen H, Smid K, Peters G, Kampinga HH: End-joining deficiency and radiosensitization induced by gemcitabine. Cancer Res 2001;61:1585–1591.

43 Blackstock A, Lesser G, Fletcher-Steede J, Case L, Tucker R, Russo S, White D, Miller A: Phase I study of twice-weekly gemcitabine and concurrent thoracic radiation for patients with locally advanced non-small-cell lung cancer. Int J Radiat Oncol Biol Phys 2001;51:1281–1289.

44 Talamonti M, Catalano P, Vaughn D, Whittington R, Beauchamp R, Berlin J, Benson A: Eastern Cooperative Oncology Group Phase I trial of protracted venous infusion fluorouracil plus weekly gemcitabine with concurrent radiation therapy in patients with locally advanced pancreas cancer: A regimen with unexpected early toxicity. J Clin Oncol 2000;18:3384–3389.

45 Pisters P, Abbruzzese J, Janjan N, Cleary K, Charnsangavej C, Crane C, Lenzi R, Vauthey N, Lee J, Abbruzzese J, Evans D: Rapid-fractionation preoperative chemoradiation, pancreaticoduodenectomy, and intraoperative radiation therapy for resectable pancreatic adenocarcinoma. J Clin Oncol 1998;16:3843–3850.

Dr. Stefan Höcht
Clinic for Radiation Oncology and Radiotherapy
Charité, Campus Benjamin Franklin
Hindenburgdamm 30, DE–12200 Berlin (Germany)
Tel. +49 30 8445 3058, Fax +49 30 8445 2991, E-Mail stefan.hoecht@medizin.fu-berlin.de

Wiegel T, Höcht S, Sternemann M, Buhr HJ, Hinkelbein W (eds): Controversies in Gastrointestinal Tumor Therapy. Front Radiat Ther Oncol. Basel, Karger, 2004, vol 38, pp 94–99

·······················

Surgical Resection of Colorectal Metastases

Sven Jonas, Armin Thelen, Christoph Benckert, Peter Neuhaus

Department of General, Visceral, and Transplantation Surgery, Charité – Campus Virchow Klinikum, Humboldt University of Berlin, Berlin, Germany

Former restrictions for the surgical resection of colorectal liver metastases have largely disappeared over the past decade. In the 1980s, more than 3 liver metastases and tumor-free resection margins of <1 cm were considered indicators of a poor prognosis [1]. However, the long-term survival rates after liver resection have markedly increased and both parameters have been shown to no longer bear any prognostic significance [2]. For 167 patients with a tumor-free liver resection margin exceeding 10 mm, 78 patients in whom it ranged from 5 to 9 mm, and 131 patients with a non-infiltrated resection margin of <4 mm, the plotted survival curves ran almost in parallel [2]. This is a phenomenon which was also seen after resection of cholangiocellular carcinomas and has also been reported in patients suffering from hepatocellular carcinomas [3]. The most likely explanation for the finding that a hepatic resection margin of at least 1 cm is too stringent a criterion for a formally curative or R0 resection is its definition according to the broadness of the resected specimen. However, the margin of the specimen forms only part of the surgical safety area around a hepatic tumor mass. In addition there are two more layers around the tumor contributing to the safety zone: the parenchymal dissection line, and a coagulation field along the resection line of the liver remnant, each measuring about 1–3 mm. Tissue destruction within the parenchymal dissection line is usually created by an ultrasound tip and the coagulation field on the remnant by infrared light. The additional resection margin can hardly be quantified and has not been considered in former retrospective analyses.

According to the current guidelines of the German Cancer Society and the German Surgical Society, contraindications with regard to the resection of colorectal liver metastasis are only given if a formally curative resection is not feasible or if lymph node metastases within the hepatoduodenal ligament or other extrahepatic tumor manifestations are present [4]. It is the current approach of many centers to confine these contraindications only to those patients in whom the extrahepatic tumor manifestations are not resectable because a considerable number of patients suffering from local recurrence of the primary tumor or pulmonary metastases have the chance of a formally curative resection on these sites as well. The significance of the lymph nodes within the hepatoduodenal ligament has been emphasized in a recent study indicating an incidence of infiltrated lymph nodes in patients with colorectal metastases of 28% [5]. Moreover, positive lymph nodes were identified as prognostic parameters in a multi-variate analysis. So far, a lymphadenectomy of the hepatoduodenal ligament has not been included in the standard surgical approach and it is still an open question whether it should be advocated to do so.

In the literature, 5-year survival rates of patients after resection of colorectal liver metastases range from 15 to 50% [2, 5–9]. Differences are supposed to be due to varying selection criteria with regard to the extent of the metastases within the liver, possible extrahepatic metastases and also the primary tumor. Other studies have reported on different time periods which may already be as long as 40 years [2]. Varying surgical approaches also have an impact on patient selection and on the results obtained. Discrimination should be made between major resections, meaning hemihepatectomies or extended resections, and minor resections. Although formal anatomic resections of one or two liver segments may be demanding surgical procedures depending on the location of the segment and possible previous hepatic resections, they are categorized as minor resections. However, minor resections frequently relate to non-anatomic wedge resections. If both procedures are technically feasible, the question whether to perform a minor or a major resection is still under debate. A contribution to this ongoing discussion is the recently published comparison of 119 patients undergoing wedge resection and 148 patients in whom formal anatomic hepatic resections were performed [10]. In this study, the rate of a positive surgical margin after hepatic wedge resections was 16% compared to the significantly lower number of 2% after formal anatomic resections. A putative advantage for more extended resections was also described in the largest study on recurrent colorectal liver metastases [11]. If the first intervention was a major resection, then this was a favorable prognostic parameter for the second hepatic resection. So far, no prospective trials comparing the safety and efficacy of minor and major liver resections for colorectal liver metastasis have been performed.

We have retrospectively reviewed the outcome of 312 patients undergoing liver resection for colorectal metastasis in our institution between 1989 and 1999. In all patients, resection of the primary colorectal cancer was categorized

Table 1. Surgical procedures in 312 patients undergoing liver resection for colorectal metastases from 1989 to 1999

	n	%
Major resections		
Hemihepatectomies	128	41
Extended resections	63	20
Trisectionectomies	19	6
Minor resections		
Wedge resections	54	17
Unisegmental resections	20	6
Segmental 2/3 resections	19	6
Plurisegmental resections	9	3

as formally curative. The diagnostic evaluation comprised total coloscopy, conventional radiography of the chest, carcinoembryonic antigen serum levels, ultrasonography and computed tomography. Intraoperatively, the abdomen was systematically examined, lymph nodes of the hepatoduodenal ligament sent for frozen section biopsy and ultrasonography repeated. The surgical procedures performed in these patients are depicted in table 1, showing 210 major resections (67%) and 102 minor resections (33%). Among the major resections, hemihepatectomies (n = 128; 41%) were the most common intervention. Extended resections and trisectionectomies were performed in 20 and 6% of the patients, respectively. Among these were also resections extending beyond a trisectionectomy, for example subtotal left hepatectomy preserving segment VII or subtotal right hepatectomy preserving parts of segments II and III. The most common intervention in the group of minor resections was wedge resection (n = 54; 17%). The postoperative 30-day mortality rate was 2% (n = 6) mainly occurring after extended liver resections. The main causes of death were cardiopulmonary and hepatic failure. The 1-, 5-, and 10-year survival rates were 82, 45, and 39%, respectively (fig. 1).

The survival rates have increased in comparison to an analysis of our own results from the early 1990s [12]. Other groups have described the same increase in survival rates when comparing different time frames. Recently, Choti et al. [6] reviewed a series of 226 patients undergoing liver resection for hepatic colorectal metastases at Johns Hopkins University. The 5-year survival rates in a cohort of 93 patients with metastases resected between 1984 and 1992 and in 133 patients resected between 1993 and 1999 were 31 and 58%, respectively; the corresponding 5-year disease-free survival rates were 14 and 28%, respectively. One criticism is the significantly shorter follow-up period in the

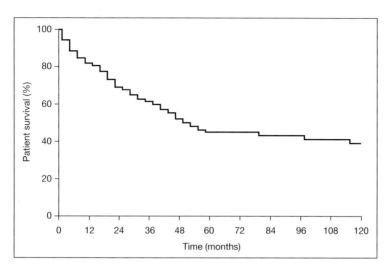

Fig. 1. Actuarial survival of 312 patients undergoing liver resection for colorectal metastases between 1989 and 1999.

latter group, resulting in a comparison of actuarial and actual patient survival. On the other hand, a variety of possible explanations for the observed trend towards an improved outcome can be considered. Advances in preoperative imaging and the implemented changes in operative technique, as well as adjuvant and neoadjuvant chemotherapeutic strategies contribute to an improvement in long-term outcome. Therefore, the authors could not identify a single causative parameter. Instead, the number of patients undergoing preoperative chemotherapy has significantly increased from 38 to 62%. The same could be observed for the number of anatomic resections which went up from 62 to 80%. In contrast, perioperative blood replacement and hospitalization time have both decreased from 2.2 to 1.0 units and 13 to 7 days, respectively, in spite of a more aggressive surgical approach. A more aggressive surgical approach also relates to the changing attitude of many institutions when confronted with recurrent disease after initial resection. Today, a significantly greater proportion of recurrences are treated with repeat surgical resection, while a nihilistic attitude is no longer justified.

Future strategies aim at increasing the number of patients with resectable liver metastases of colorectal cancer from a figure which is currently estimated to range from 20–25 up to 30–35%. These strategies aim at an downstaging, increasing the resectable liver volume or an combination of different strategies, for example the combination of liver resection and in situ tumor ablation. This combination is intraoperatively most frequently performed using radio-frequency tumor ablation. Thus, multiple metastases which may not be completely resected can be left in the remnant liver tissue and destroyed locally. The main disadvantage of in situ tumor ablation is the histologically uncontrollable result. Even tumor necrosis of 99.99%, which is not detectable by current diagnostic procedures, results in a survival of 10^6 vital tumor cells if the given tumor volume was, for example, $10 \, cm^3$ equaling 10^{10} tumor cells. Moreover, the number and size of metastases which can be treated with in situ ablation methods are limited to patients with rather small metastases.

Downstaging protocols are largely restricted to neoadjuvant chemotherapy regimens. The largest experience originates from Bismuth et al. [13]. In this study of 330 patients in whom the liver metastases were considered as non-resectable, 53 finally underwent liver resection after combination chemotherapy using Oxaliplatin, 5-FU and folinic acid. The 5-year survival rate in this group was 40% and did not differ from patients with primarily resectable metastases. Patients with the largest benefit were those suffering from ill-located and large tumor nodules.

In contrast to downstaging, resectability can also be achieved by extending the total resectable liver volume. The most promising approach is unilateral portal vein embolization, which was described for bile duct cancers in 1990 by Makuuchi et al. [14] and for colorectal liver metastases in 2000 by Azoulay et al. [15]. In the latter study, 30 patients with non-resectable colorectal metastases were included. The anticipated postoperatively remaining liver parenchyma was calculated to be less than 40% of the total liver volume by CT volumetry. Unilateral portal vein embolization resulted in a significant increase in the putative remaining parenchyma from 26 to 37%. A liver resection was hence performed in 19 patients (63%) with a 5-year survival rate of 40%.

In conclusion a formally curative resection is the most relevant prognostic parameter in patients suffering from colorectal liver metastases. A tumor-free margin of <1 cm and the number of metastases do not indicate an impaired prognosis. While the combination of surgical resection and in situ ablation may increase the number of long-term survivors, local tumor control is still a problem after an in situ ablation. Multimodal strategies may increase the number of resectable patients from 20–25% to 30–35%. Therefore, the treatment of patients with colorectal liver metastases should only be performed if the entire multimodal armamentarium is available.

References

1   Ekberg H, Tranberg KG, Andersson R, Lundstedt C, Hagerstrand I, Ranstam J, Bengmark S: Determinants of survival in liver resection for colorectal secondaries. Br J Surg 1986;73: 727–731.

2   Scheele J, Altendorf-Hofmann A, Stangl R, Schmidt K: Surgical resection of colorectal liver metastases: Gold standard for solitary and radically resectable lesions (in German). Swiss Surg 1996(suppl 4):4–17.

3   Poon RT, Fan ST, Lo CM, Ng IO, Liu CL, Lam CM, Wong J: Improving survival results after resection of hepatocellular carcinoma: A prospective study of 377 patients over 10 years. Ann Surg 2001;234:63–70.

4   Diagnostik und Therapie von Lebermetastasen; in Junginger Th, Hossfeld DK, Müller R-P (Hrsg): Leitlinien zur Diagnostik und Therapie von Tumoren des Gastrointestinaltrakts und der Schilddrüse. Deutsche Gesellschaft für Chirurgie/Deutsche Krebsgesellschaft e.V. Stuttgart, Demeter/Thieme, 1999, pp 87–90.

5   Beckurts KT, Holscher AH, Thorban S, Bollschweiler E, Siewert JR: Significance of lymph node involvement at the hepatic hilum in the resection of colorectal liver metastases. Br J Surg 1997;84:1081–1084.

6   Choti MA, Sitzmann JV, Tiburi MF, Sumetchotimetha W, Rangsin R, Schulick RD, Lillemoe KD, Yeo CJ, Cameron JL: Trends in long-term survival following liver resection for hepatic colorectal metastases. Ann Surg 2002;235:759–766.

7   Fong Y, Fortner J, Sun RL, Brennan MF, Blumgart LH: Clinical score for predicting recurrence after hepatic resection for metastatic colorectal cancer: Analysis of 1001 consecutive cases. Ann Surg 1999;230:309–318.

8   Jenkins LT, Millikan KW, Bines SD, Staren ED, Doolas A: Hepatic resection for metastatic colorectal cancer. Am Surg 1997;63:605–610.

9   Gayowski TJ, Iwatsuki S, Madariaga JR, Selby R, Todo S, Irish W, Starzl TE: Experience in hepatic resection for metastatic colorectal cancer: Analysis of clinical and pathologic risk factors. Surgery 1994;116:703–710.

10 DeMatteo RP, Palese C, Jarnagin WR, Sun RL, Blumgart LH, Fong Y: Anatomic segmental hepatic resection is superior to wedge resection as an oncologic operation for colorectal liver metastases. J Gastrointest Surg 2000;4:178–184.

11 Scheele J, Stangl R, Schmidt K, Altendorf-Hofmann A: Das Tumorrezidiv nach R0-Resektion colorectaler Lebermetastasen. Häufigkeit, Resektabilität und Prognose. Chirurg 1995;66:965–973.

12 Jonas S, Kling N, Bechstein WO, Kley C, Rayes N, Schumacher G, Neuhaus P: Minor versus major hepatic resections for colorectal metastases. Br J Surg 1994;81(suppl):87.

13 Bismuth H, Adam R, Lévi F, Farabos C, Waechter F, Castaing D, Majno P, Engerran L: Resection of nonresectable liver metastases from colorectal cancer after neoadjuvant chemotherapy. Ann Surg 1996;224:509–520.

14 Makuuchi M, Thai BL, Takayasu K, Takayama T, Kosuge T, Gunven P, Yamazaki S, Hasegawa H, Ozaki H: Preoperative portal embolization to increase safety of major hepatectomy for hilar bile duct carcinoma: A preliminary report. Surgery 1990;107:521–527.

15 Azoulay D, Castaing D, Smail A, Adam R, Cailliez V, Laurent A, Lemoine A, Bismuth H: Resection of nonresectable liver metastases from colorectal cancer after percutaneous portal vein embolization. Ann Surg 2000;231:480–486.

Priv.-Doz. Dr. Sven Jonas
Department of General, Visceral, and Transplantation Surgery
Charité, Campus Virchow, Humboldt University of Berlin
Augustenburger Platz 1, DE–13353 Berlin (Germany)
Tel. +49 30 450 552603, Fax +49 30 450 552900, E-Mail sven.jonas@charite.de

Wiegel T, Höcht S, Sternemann M, Buhr HJ, Hinkelbein W (eds): Controversies in Gastrointestinal
Tumor Therapy. Front Radiat Ther Oncol. Basel, Karger, 2004, vol 38, pp 100–105

....

Stereotactic Radiation Therapy of Liver Metastases: Update of the Initial Phase-I/II Trial

Klaus K. Herfarth, J. Debus, M. Wannenmacher

Division of Radiation Oncology, German Cancer Research Center,
Heidelberg, and Department of Radiation Oncology,
University of Heidelberg, Heidelberg, Germany

The first report of successful radiation therapy of liver metastases was
published in 1954. Phillips et al. [1] reported on the palliative effect in patients
with symptomatic liver metastases. Whole liver radiation therapy is still an
indication for palliation in case of pain and bile stasis in a metastatic liver.
However, no curative doses can be applied due to the radiosensitivity of the
liver tissue. Radiation-induced liver disease is characterized by ascites, jaundice, abdominal girth and an elevation in liver enzymes, especially alkaline
phosphatase [2]. The incidence of radiation-induced liver disease increases for
doses above 30 Gy when fractionation is used [3]. By using a 3-dimensional
treatment plan, sufficient sparing of liver tissue is possible and higher doses can
be applied to parts of the liver [4]. The Ann Arbor Group published several trials
using 3-dimensional conformal radiotherapy in combination with intra-arterial
chemotherapy in the treatment of liver malignancies [5–8]. However, safety
margins of 1–2.5 cm around the clinical target volume are still necessary [6].
Further reduction of the safety margin is the aim of a stereotactic treatment
approach. Lax et al. [9] and Blomgren et al. [10, 11] published the first steps in
extracranial stereotactic radiation therapy. They developed a stereotactic body
frame which allows precise positioning of the patient. We developed our own
stereotactic frame which allows fixation using a vacuum pillow with an abdominal compression device (single-dose therapy of liver and lung tumors) or a
rigid body cast (fractionated stereotactic therapy for paraspinal or pelvic
tumors) [12–14].

The precision of our system in combination with a vacuum pillow was tested for liver tumors in 36 consecutive patients treated with stereotactic single-dose radiation therapy. Using the quantitative evaluation of bony landmarks, a mean set-up error of 1.8 mm latero-lateral and 1.9 mm anterior-posterior with standard deviations of 1.1 and 0.6 mm, respectively, could be achieved (updated data from Herfarth et al. [13]). However, at least one correction of patient positioning had to be performed in 61% (22/36) cases to achieve this accuracy. The quantitative evaluation of the positioning of the treated liver tumors resulted in a comparable results: the mean set-up error in the transversal plane was 2.3 mm with a standard deviation of 1.6 and 1.9 mm in the latero-lateral and anterior-posterior direction, respectively. The deviation in the cranio-caudal direction was greater (3.4 ± 2.5 mm) due to breathing movements (updated data from Herfarth et al. [13]). The movement of the diaphragm was median 7 mm with a maximum of 13 mm measured under fluoroscopy (updated data from Herfarth et al. [13]).

Based on these data, we concluded that at least a safety margin of 6 mm should be necessary around the clinical target volume in the transversal plane. The safety margin in the cranio-caudal direction should be at least 10 mm. Our data are comparable with the results of others using similar approaches [10, 15].

First clinical results of stereotactic radiation therapy of liver malignancies were published by Blomgren et al. [10] in 1995 with an update of their data in 1998 [11]. Treating 21 patients with liver tumors, they achieved a crude local tumor control of 95% with a mean follow-up of 9.6 months [11]. This group favored a hypofractionated approach since they had had a WHO grade-V morbidity after single-dose treatment. This happened at the start of their studies after therapy of a patient with a large tumor in a cirrhotic liver.

Nevertheless, based on our experience with single-dose radiotherapy in the treatment of brain metastases [16], we decided to transform the same concept to the body stem.

A phase-I/II study was initiated in 1997 to evaluate the feasibility, the morbidity and the clinical outcome of stereotactic single-dose radiation therapy of inoperable liver tumors. The ethics committee of the University of Heidelberg approved the study. It included patients with a maximum of 3 inoperable liver metastases. The tumors did not have to be adjacent to bowel structures. The size of the tumors was limited to 6 cm. Patients with insufficient liver function were excluded. Thirty-seven patients with a total of 60 liver tumors entered this trial. The median age was 61 (range 37–84) years. Four patients had primary liver cancers (1 hepatocellular carcinoma and 3 cholangiocellular carcinoma). The other patients had metastases from colorectal cancers (n = 18), breast cancer (n = 10) and other primary cancers. The median volume of the tumors was 10 (range 1–132) ml. Other manifestations of the tumors at the time of treatment were known in 12 patients. Treatment details have been published elsewhere [17]. Shortly, the dose was applied using 5–10 conformal beams. The dose was escalated from 14 Gy/isocenter (80% isodose surrounding the planning target volume) to 26 Gy/isocenter. Before each treatment, the correct position of the target in the stereotactic frame was verified using a control CT. Set-up changes were made whenever necessary.

All patients were followed on a regular basis. Whenever possible the follow-up examination were performed at the German Cancer Research Center. The first follow-up examination was 5–10 weeks after therapy. Following appointments were every 3–5 months. Two patients could not be followed. These patients showed rapid systemic tumor progression with a strongly reduced performance status. Follow-up examination included a CT scan, clinical examination and biochemical examinations. Up to March 2002, the mean follow-up time was 15.1 months with a maximum of 50.6 months. Here, we present the updated data of our earlier published evaluation [17].

There were no major morbidities observed after the treatment. The only side effects were nausea, hiccup and fever. There was no morbidity grade of more than 2 (common toxicity criteria). There were also no significant changes in liver enzyme concentrations. No radiation-induced liver disease was observed. Radiologically, there was a focal radiation reaction visible in the liver. This radiation reaction will be characterized in detail elsewhere.

A clinical response to the therapy could be observed in all but 1 patient. Of the 55 tumors with follow-up, 22 showed stable disease, 28 partial response and 4 complete response at the first follow-up examination. After 6 months, 14% (6/44) of the tumors showed stable disease, 48% (21/44) partial response, 18% (8/44) complete response, and 9 tumors demonstrated local failure. Actuarial local tumor control was 68% at 18 months for all patients. However, it was 81% for patients treated at phase II after the initial dose escalation and the optimization of patients positioning (fig. 1). Different tumor histologies (colorectal cancer and breast cancer) had no statistically different local tumor control rates. There was also no statistically significant difference if only 1 tumor (n = 24) or more than 1 tumor was treated (n = 11). Tumor volume also did not influence local tumor control in the patients treated in phase II: 32 tumors with <15 ml showed an actuarial local tumor control of 85% at 18 months, and 17 larger tumors had a tumor control probability of 80% at this time.

Additional chemotherapy was given in 13 of the phase-II patients. This was done either at the time of treatment (n = 5) or during further follow-up (n = 8). Censoring the patients at the start of chemotherapy, the actuarial local tumor control was 78% at 18 months. Therefore, we conclude that the results of the radiation treatment were not significantly influenced by the additional chemotherapy.

The median survival of all patients has been 25 months, and it has been 27 months for the phase-II patients. In the latter group, there was a significant

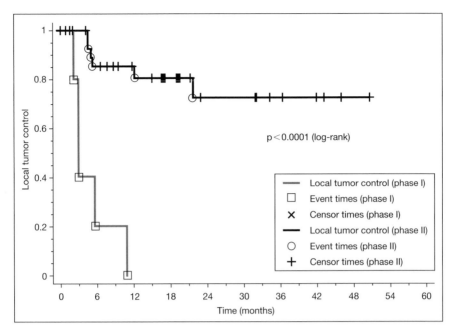

Fig. 1. Actuarial local tumor control after 37 patient treatments. The patients treated during phase II show a significantly better survival.

survival benefit for those patients who did not show additional tumor manifestations at the time of treatment (median survival 35.8 vs. 11.3 months; fig. 2).

Our data show that stereotactic single-dose radiation therapy is feasible without major side effects. The basis for sufficient and safe therapy is reliable positioning of the patient. A vacuum pillow and an abdominal compression device seem to be suitable to achieve accurate positioning. However, a control CT should be performed before each treatment to ensure the correct positioning and prompt changes if necessary. The effect of radiation seems to be independent of additional chemotherapy, histology or size of the tumor. However, patient numbers are too small to draw definitive conclusions about influencing parameters. The results are comparable with those of other groups using a hypofractionated approach. Wulf et al. [18] reported an actuarial local tumor control rate of 76% after 72 months in 23 patients treated with 3 × 10 Gy to the surrounding 65% isodose.

The major advantage compared to other local ablation methods is the non-invasiveness of this approach. Also centrally located liver lesions can be treated without the risk of vessel injury or a heat shift the periphery as is described for thermo-ablative procedures [19, 20].

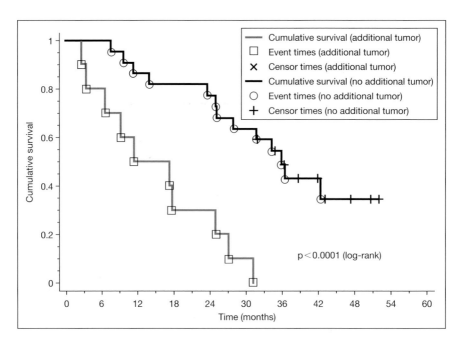

Fig. 2. Actuarial overall survival of 35 patients treated during phase II. Patients without additional tumor show a significantly better survival with a median survival of 36 months.

For further evaluation of this method, a multi-center phase-III trial has been initiated. This trial should compare the two published principles of stereotactic radiation therapy in the treatment of liver metastases: single-dose irradiation with a homogenous dose concept (80% isodose surrounding the planned target volume) versus hypofractionation using 3 fractions with an inhomogenous dose concept (65% isodose surrounding the planned target volume). The trial has been approved by the German Cancer Society. Results of this trial will confirm the effectiveness of stereotactic radiation therapy of liver metastases.

References

1   Phillips R, Karnofsky DA, Hamilton LD, Nickson JJ: Roentgen therapy of hepatic metastases. Am J Roentgenol Rad Ther Nucl Med 1954;71:826–834.
2   Lawrence TS, Robertson JM, Anscher MS, Jirtle RL, Ensminger WD, Fajardo LF: Hepatic toxicity resulting from cancer treatment. Int J Radiat Oncol Biol Phys 1995;31:1237–1248.
3   Russell AH, Clyde C, Wasserman TH, Turner SS, Rotman M: Accelerated hyperfractionated hepatic irradiation in the management of patients with liver metastases: Results of the RTOG dose escalating protocol. Int J Radiat Oncol Biol Phys 1993;27:117–123.

4   Dawson LA, Ten Haken RK, Lawrence TS: Partial irradiation of the liver. Semin Radiat Oncol 2001;11:240–246.

5   Robertson JM, Lawrence TS, Dworzanin LM, Andrews JC, Walker S, Kessler ML, DuRoss DJ, Ensminger WD: Treatment of primary hepatobiliary cancers with conformal radiation therapy and regional chemotherapy. J Clin Oncol 1993;11:1286–1293.

6   Robertson JM, Lawrence TS, Walker S, Kessler ML, Andrews JC, Ensminger WD: The treatment of colorectal liver metastases with conformal radiation therapy and regional chemotherapy. Int J Radiat Oncol Biol Phys 1995;32:445–450.

7   Robertson JM, McGinn CJ, Walker S, Marx MV, Kessler ML, Ensminger WD, Lawrence TS: A phase I trial of hepatic arterial bromodeoxyuridine and conformal radiation therapy for patients with primary hepatobiliary cancers or colorectal liver metastases. Int J Radiat Oncol Biol Phys 1997;39:1087–1092.

8   Dawson LA, McGinn CJ, Normolle D, Ten Haken RK, Walker S, Ensminger W, Lawrence TS: Escalated focal liver radiation and concurrent hepatic artery fluorodeoxyuridine for unresectable intrahepatic malignancies. J Clin Oncol 2000;18:2210–2218.

9   Lax I, Blomgren H, Näslund I, Svanström R: Stereotactic radiotherapy of malignancies in the abdomen. Acta Oncol 1994;33:677–683.

10 Blomgren H, Lax I, Näslund I, Svanström R: Stereotactic high dose fraction radiation therapy of extracranial tumors using an accelerator. Acta Oncol 1995;34:861–870.

11 Blomgren H, Lax I, Göranson H, Kræpelien T, Nilsson B, Näslund I, Svanström R, Tilikidis A: Radiosurgery for tumors in the body: Clinical experience using a new method. J Radiosurg 1998;1:63–74.

12 Lohr F, Debus J, Frank C, Herfarth K, Pastyr O, Rhein B, Bahner ML, Schlegel W, Wannenmacher M: Noninvasive patient fixation for extracranial stereotactic radiotherapy. Int J Radiat Oncol Biol Phys 1999;45:521–527.

13 Herfarth KK, Debus J, Lohr F, Bahner ML, Fritz P, Höss A, Schlegel W, Wannenmacher M: Extracranial stereotactic radiation therapy: Set-up accuracy of patients treated for liver metastases. Int J Radiat Oncol Biol Phys 2000;46:329–335.

14 Herfarth KK, Pirzkall A, Lohr F, Schulz-Ertner D, Spoo J, Bahner ML, Pastyr O, Debus J: Erste Erfahrungen mit einem nicht-invasiven Patientenfixierungssystem für die stereotaktische Strahlentherapie der Prostata. Strahlenther Onkol 2000;176:217–222.

15 Wulf J, Hädinger U, Oppitz U, Olshausen B, Flentje M: Stereotactic radiotherapy of extracranial targets: CT-simulation and accuracy of treatment in the stereotactic body frame. Radiother Oncol 2000;57:225–236.

16 Pirzkall A, Debus J, Lohr F, Fuss M, Rhein B, Engenhart-Cabillic R, Wannenmacher M: Radiosurgery alone or in combination with whole-brain radiotherapy for brain metastases. J Clin Oncol 1998;16:3563–3569.

17 Herfarth KK, Debus J, Lohr F, Bahner ML, Rhein B, Fritz P, Höss A, Schlegel W, Wannenmacher MF: Stereotactic single dose radiation therapy of liver tumors: Results of a phase I/II trial. J Clin Oncol 2001;19:164–170.

18 Wulf J, Hädinger U, Oppitz U, Thiele W, Ness-Dourdoumas R, Flentje M: Stereotactic radiotherapy of targets in the lung and liver. Strahlenther Onkol 2001;177:645–655.

19 Helmberger T, Holzknecht N, Schöpf U, Kulinna C, Rau H, Stäbler A, Reiser M: Radiofrequenzablation von Lebermetastasen. Radiologe 2001;41:69–76.

20 Vogl T, Mack M, Straub R, Zangos S, Woitaschek D, Eichler K, Engelmann K: Thermische Ablation von Lebermetastasen. Radiologe 2001;41:49–55.

Klaus K. Herfarth, MD
Division Radiation Oncology, E0500
INF 280, DE–69120 Heidelberg (Germany)
Tel. +49 6221 422587, Fax +49 6221 422514, E-Mail k.herfarth@dkfz.de

Wiegel T, Höcht S, Sternemann M, Buhr HJ, Hinkelbein W (eds): Controversies in Gastrointestinal
Tumor Therapy. Front Radiat Ther Oncol. Basel, Karger, 2004, vol 38, pp 106–121

....

Laser-Induced Thermotherapy of Liver Metastases

J.-P. Ritz[a], *C. Isbert*[a], *A. Roggan*[b], *H.J. Buhr*[a], *C.-T. Germer*[a]

[a] Department for General, Vascular and Thoracic Surgery, and
[b] Institute for Medical Physics and Laser Medicine, Charité Medical
University Berlin, Campus Benjamin Franklin, Berlin, Germany

Laser-induced thermotherapy (LITT), first described by Bown [1] in 1983, is an effective, minimally invasive treatment strategy for the local destruction of tumors with the preservation of healthy surrounding tissue. Laser light at high power levels is guided through flexible light waveguides into the target tissue. By photon absorption temperatures in the range 55–150°C are achieved, resulting in substantial tissue coagulation, subsequent cell death and tissue necrosis. The procedure can be realized both percutaneously and laparoscopically as well as in open surgery [2]. In contrast to surgical procedures, the treated tissue volume remains in situ after its destruction. Therefore, LITT is also termed an in situ ablation technique (fig.1). The basic idea to use heat for the destruction of pathological tissue was already known as early as 1700 BC. Breast tumors were reported to have been treated with a red-hot iron tip [3]. The first quantitative in vivo study on thermal tissue damage was performed by Henriques and Moritz [4] in 1947. After development of the first clinical laser systems, thermal ablation was revived as a method in the early 1980s. First applications of LITT, also called laser-induced coagulation, interstitial laser thermotherapy or interstitial laser photocoagulation, were focused on brain tumors, liver tumors and the vascular system. Later the indication was extended to the treatment of benign prostatic hyperplasia, tumors of the head and neck region, gynecologic and breast tumors.

Most experience with LITT has been gained with liver metastases of colorectal carcinomas. Here in many cases metastatic spread is initially limited to the liver and only about 30% of the patients can be considered for potentially

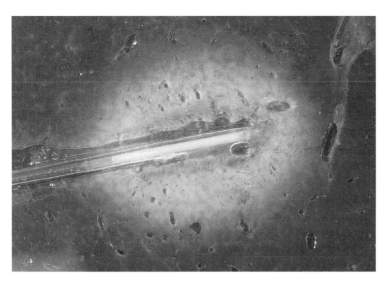

Fig. 1. Laser-induced thermotherapy in porcine liver.

curative surgery based on their prognostic factors [5]. Thus, alternative treatment concepts are needed for the majority of patients. Due to the high radiosensitivity of the liver parenchyma, curative treatment of liver metastases is not possible by percutaneous radiation as it requires a relatively high dose of 50–60 Gy [6]. Moreover, systemic or local chemotherapy of liver metastases has a poor response with median survival rates of 11.1–12.7 months [7, 8]. By way of comparison, surgical resection has a median survival rate of 27–46 months [9]. In the largest LITT study performed so far, Vogl et al. [10] obtained a mean cumulative survival rate of more than 40 months in patients with colorectal liver metastases. The enormous potential of LITT becomes evident when it is considered that these patients were unable to undergo resection because of their poor prognostic factors.

Laser Systems and Laser–Tissue Interaction

The temporal course of the temperature distribution during local heating of biological tissue is determined by two processes: the local development of heat and the simultaneous dissipation and conduction of thermal energy. Although the first process is determined by the light distribution and the absorption properties of the target tissue, the second process depends not only on heat conduction and local blood perfusion but also metabolic changes and phase transitions

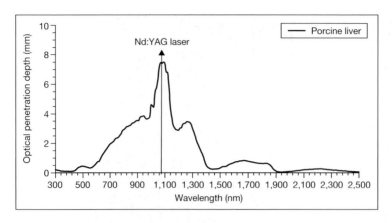

Fig. 2. Optical penetration depth in porcine liver, calculated from the optical parameter absorption, scattering and scattering phase function.

[11, 12]. The first question to be answered to ensure safe and reproducible application of LITT is which laser wavelength is best suited for the treatment. Most applications of LITT are related to the treatment of targets from 1 to >5 cm in diameter. It is therefore evident that a laser wavelength with a high penetration depth is the one most suited to treat large volumes, using a moderate temperature gradient with a minimum risk of thermal damage to the application system. It is known from investigation of the optical tissue parameters that the wavelength region with maximum optical penetration, the so-called 'optical window', ranges from approximately 800 to 1,100 nm [13]. Figure 2 shows the optical penetration depth of liver tissue calculated from its optical parameters (absorption, scattering and scattering phase function), demonstrating the optical window with a penetration depth of about 8 mm at 1,070 nm [14]. Consequently, the Nd:YAG laser at 1,064 nm is the laser which is most often applied in LITT [15]. Typical laser powers for LITT range from 5 to 30 W in continuous wave mode, mainly depending on the preferred volume of destruction and the applicator system used (see below).

As has already been mentioned, LITT is frequently applied in order to destroy large tumors. Bearing in mind that the optical penetration depth of most target tissues is in the range of 1 cm at 1,064 nm, relatively long exposure times are required, using heat conduction as an additional physical mechanism to increase thermal lesion size. The typical speed of a thermal front in bulk tissue can be estimated to be as follows [16]:

 1 mm: 1 s
 10 mm: 100 s
 30 mm: 1,000 s

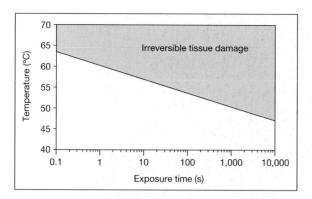

Fig. 3. Laser–tissue interaction as a function of temperature.

In addition to optical penetration and heat conduction, the temporal course of interstitial thermotherapy also depends on the local blood perfusion as a cooling mechanism [12]. Consequently, relevant tumor sizes require exposure periods of 10–30 min to achieve total destruction of pathologic tissue.

The high temperatures reached during LITT lead to substantial coagulation of tissue in which the spatial configuration of protein molecules is modified. Enzyme denaturation and inhibition of protein synthesis result in membrane defects with subsequent edema formation and cell death as a direct consequence [17]. In this way LITT differs fundamentally from classic hyperthermia which aims at temperatures of around 43.5°C and attempts to destroy tumor cells through their higher thermal sensitivity. However, a margin surrounding the target tissue with temperatures between 42 and 50°C is also found during LITT. Here adjuvant hyperthermal effects can be observed. Figure 3 shows the laser–tissue interaction as a function of the maximum temperature [18]. It can be seen that a temperature of 55°C requires approximately 30 s to reach irreversible tissue damage. This also explains why exposure periods for LITT are longer than usual in high power laser applications.

Laser Applicators

The first applications of interstitial laser coagulation were conducted using the so-called 'bare fiber'. The advantage of the bare fiber is its small diameter which ranges from 400 to 600 μm allowing it to be easily introduced into the target tissue using hollow puncture needles. This technique has been used frequently in the treatment of congenital vascular malformations in children [19]. But there is one significant drawback to the bare fiber: all laser energy must be

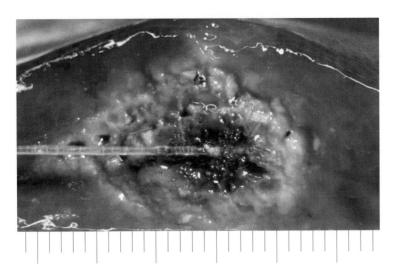

Fig. 4. Tissue charring using a bare fiber interstitially (Nd:YAG laser, 5 W, 5 min, porcine liver).

transmitted through the distal fiber area which is smaller than $0.3\,mm^2$ for a 600-μm fiber. This leads to power densities of approximately $1\,kW/cm^2$ at a laser power of only 3 W, resulting in temperatures above 100°C within a few seconds of exposure. Consequently charring of the tissue is the outcome with the bare fiber, when using high laser powers or the prolonged exposure periods necessary for efficient tumor treatment. This means that the radiation can no longer penetrate the carbonized tissue and the maximum coagulation diameter is limited to about 1 cm (fig. 4).

As a result, further efforts have been made to produce larger lesions and reduce the tendency to char [20, 21]. The most recent generation of application systems for LITT are called scattering applicators or diffusing tips (fig. 5). Laser radiation is laterally coupled out of the fiber over an active length of up to 3 cm by means of scattering [22, 23]. The fiber is chemically etched (frosted), the tip is also protected by a glass cap, which is 1 mm in diameter and 20–40 mm in length. The main advantage of this technique is that the tip can be guided through flexible endoscopes and catheters without the risk of mechanical damage.

Puncture Equipment and Puncture Control

Most LITT applications are done with a minimally invasive intention. This means that the laser fibers are placed percutaneously utilizing a monitored

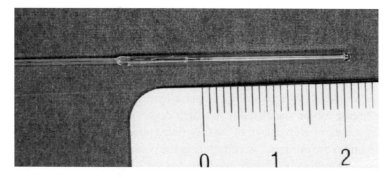

Fig. 5. Diffuser tip applicator/scattering applicator (diameter 1.0 mm).

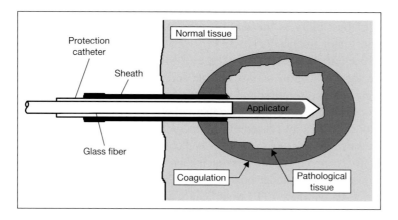

Fig. 6. LITT configuration of laser fiber, applicator, protection catheter, and sheath.

puncture procedure. As has already been mentioned, scattering applicators are positioned within the target tissue using a distally closed, flexible protection catheter. This requires a multi-step puncture procedure (Seldinger technique) in order to achieve optimal catheter position as shown in figure 6. Optimized puncture and application kits have been developed for this purpose [22]. The first step is the puncture of the target tissue using a hollow needle (18 gauge). This allows insertion of a flexible guide wire (0.089 cm). The guide wire allows the sheath/dilatator combination (7 french) to be introduced into the target. The protection catheter (6 french) can now be pushed through the sheath after removal of the guide wire and mandrin. The sheath must be finally withdrawn by 4 cm to ensure free radiation of the distal catheter region. Now the scattering applicator can be introduced into the catheter and fixed at the proximal end to prevent dislocation during treatment. It is evident that the Seldinger procedure requires precise monitoring to visualize not only target position and puncture direction but also to avoid damage to sensitive structures (vessels, colon) in the direction of the puncture. In practice, there are three methods frequently used for LITT [24].

(1) The best resolution is given by computer tomography (CT). The tumor and puncture needle can be visualized with a high degree of contrast to other tissues. However, a minor disadvantage of the CT-guided puncture is that only transverse representations are available, which restricts the possible puncture direction.

(2) A simple handling procedure can be achieved if ultrasound imaging is used for puncture control. Each angle between the scanner and puncture needle can be applied and the needle has a significant contrast to the tissue. But problems may arise if the target is located directly near air-filled structures and/or below bones (e.g. in the cranial part of the liver).

(3) A third possibility is the use of open magnetic resonance imaging (MRI). Here the tumor and needle are easy to see and the imaged planes can be maintained at each angle [25]. However, use of MR-compatible equipment is necessary and the application of fast on-line sequences during the puncture process reduces spatial resolution and increases noise. Nevertheless, MRI can also be used for on-line monitoring of the thermal effects without repositioning the patient after the puncture procedure. So the whole LITT treatment can be done using the same monitoring system throughout.

Apart from the percutaneous approach there are also indications for a LITT procedure carried out under open surgery [2]. One example is the treatment of liver metastases where LITT treatment of a single metastasis may bring the patient into a resectable situation for the residual liver metastases. Figure 7 shows the typical intra-operative situation with ultrasound-guided puncture control, introduced catheter and laser applicator and enclosed ligamentum hepatoduodenale.

Methods for Efficiency Improvement

The maximum diameter of thermal necrosis is limited to about 3 cm using a scattering applicator and standard protection catheters. However, under the aspect of an oncological treatment concept, a safety margin of 5–10 mm is always required around a malignant tumor, either during surgical resection or if an in situ ablation technique is applied. Consequently, the maximum diameter for oncological LITT treatments was limited to about 2 cm. Nevertheless, most tumors indicated for LITT have a larger diameter so that various techniques have been developed in order to increase the maximum lesion size.

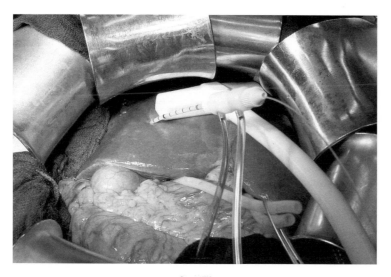

Fig. 7. Typical situs during LITT in open surgery.

A first step towards attaining larger coagulation volumes was the development of a modified protection catheter [22, 26]. Introduction of a second tube into the catheter has enabled coaxial flow of a cooling liquid to be realized (fig. 8). Saline solution at room temperature and a flow rate of 60 ml/min is normally used as the cooling liquid. Maximum coagulation diameters of up to 5 cm were measured in an in vivo porcine liver model with interrupted blood perfusion. By way of conclusion, the cooled catheter can be regarded as a significant improvement and is one which is currently applied in 90% of all LITT procedures.

A further possibility of increasing the treatment efficiency is multiple ablation of the target region. If the tumor shape differs significantly from a sphere, a second application, after moderate withdrawal of the applicator, may increase the lesion size and create an ellipsoidal shape. However, a much more efficient method is the simultaneous multiple application procedure. Up to five cooled scattering applicators can be positioned within one tumor and all applicators are activated synchronously. The main advantage is the superposition of the various temperature fields produced by the single applicators which considerably increases the efficiency compared to a asynchronous thermal ablation with the same number of applicators. Utilizing this technique, tumor sizes of up to 5 cm can be included in a LITT protocol.

In addition, a second mechanism can be used to improve the efficiency of LITT. As mentioned before, the flow of blood removes a considerable amount of thermal energy from the target region [12]. This energy is therefore no longer

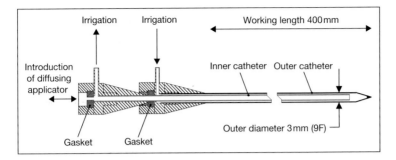

Fig. 8. Cooled protection catheter for the application of high laser powers.

available for thermal coagulation. Consequently, interruption of the blood supply will increase the efficiency significantly. However, this procedure can only be done in a few organs but has been demonstrated for the liver in various ways [2]. It is possible to perform a Pringle maneuver during open surgery LITT, i.e. temporal interruption of the liver blood supply at the ligamentum hepatoduodenale for a period of up to 45 min. This course of action has been proven to be nearly as effective as using three applicators simultaneously without interruption of the blood supply [12]. Current research results show that the combination of LITT with temporary microembolization by microspheres made of starch also increases the efficiency and especially the therapeutic safety in the margin of the thermal lesion [27, 28]. The microspheres are directly injected into the arteria hepatica via a catheter a few minutes before laser therapy. This procedure can also be selected if a percutaneous approach is planned and the introduction of a liver catheter can be tolerated by the patient. After about an hour the spheres dissolve without further intervention [29].

Therapy Planning

As demonstrated, the modern technical prerequisites for LITT provide safe and effective thermal destruction of tumors ranging up to 5 cm in diameter. However, due to the dynamic behavior of the optical and thermal tissue parameters, an accurate prediction of the final thermal necrosis is difficult, especially if the multiple applicator technique is applied. Therefore, a numerical model has been developed to calculate the laser–tissue interaction and to compute optimal power settings and geometric configurations in advance of treatment [14, 30, 31]. However, calculating laser-induced thermal tissue reactions is a complex task which requires the compilation of different physical processes while considering variable parameters: (1) calculation of the radiative transport

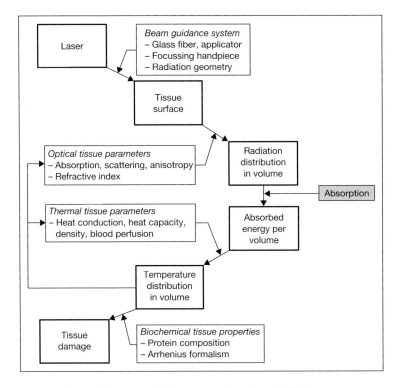

Fig. 9. Dosimetry model for therapy planning of LITT.

in scattering and absorbing media; (2) calculation of heat transfer by heat conduction and via the blood flow, and (3) calculation of the thermal tissue damage.

The dosimetry model applied to high precision calculations is given in figure 9, demonstrating the numerous parameters which depend dynamically on the actual tissue state. Converting the model for the computer first requires the physical description of the processes involved, as well as the selection of suitable mathematical methods for their implementation in a radiation planning system. In this context, a decisive requirement is complete three-dimensionality for the adequate calculation of procedures such as multiple puncture of a tumor. Therefore, the region of interest containing the tumor is separated into so-called 'volume elements' (voxels) with a typical dimension of 1 mm. Each voxel carries its own set of physical parameters, the required overall dimension of the region of interest depends on tumor extent and target organ, but is typically set to 10 cm. The simulation is operated using input menus in which the required data are entered for practically every interstitial application with various applicator

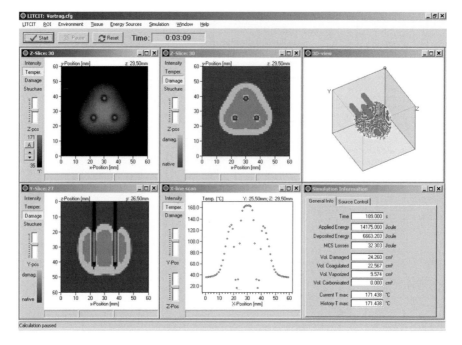

Fig. 10. Multi-window display of a computer model for therapy planning of LITT (Laser- und Medizin-Technologie Berlin, Germany).

types (scattering applicators, bare fiber, etc.). The optical and thermal parameters for a specific tissue are either taken from a data base or entered freely. Various diagrams can be selected during the simulation which give information on the current course of the therapy (fig. 10).

Therapy Control

Before the laser applicators can be introduced into the protective catheter, a power control should be carried out using a special power meter with an integrating sphere. The integrating sphere should be equipped with a sterile insertion and be able to collect all laser light emitted from the scattering applicators. A power check is recommended because fiber lengths of up to 12 m are routinely used in the clinic in order to position the laser system outside the magnetic field if MRI is used for therapy control. Hence significant losses or fiber damage may be missed if no power control is carried out. Although laser applicators with well-known characteristics are used and recent models for radiation planning show a high degree of accuracy, adequate therapy control is indispensable during laser therapy because the tissue reaction is not subject to direct visual inspection.

In the search for a suitable monitoring procedure, sonography was initially given special attention because of its low costs, high sensitivity in detecting focal liver lesions, and high availability. In percutaneous LITT on healthy pig livers, Dachman et al. [32] correlated in vivo sonographic with histomorphological findings. The authors detected a diffusely echo-rich area with numerous gas bubbles at the distal fiber end during laser exposure. However, the approximate extension of the thermally damaged tissue could only be evaluated 5–10 min after laser application. Other authors also observed massive bubble formation during on-line sonography [2, 33, 34]. The resultant hyper-reflexive shadow made it extremely difficult to evaluate the full extent of the induced lesion [19]. In conclusion, sonography must be seen as a helpful tool to aid the puncture process, but online estimation of the amount of tissue destruction is limited by significant artifacts.

The gold standard for high precision on-line monitoring of laser coagulation is still MRI. Despite its high technical expenditure, the heated tissue shows a significant loss in signal intensity so that a direct estimation of the laser–tissue interaction is possible [35, 36]. The basic concept of using MRI for thermometry is the fact that various parameters, such as the relaxation times (T1, T2) and the chemical shift, strongly depend on tissue temperature. Therefore, special modes have been developed for clinical LITT protocols, most of them using thermo-sensitive T1-weighted sequences because they are less sensitive to moving artifacts, are widely available, and data acquisition is relatively fast. Special FLASH and Turbo-FLASH sequences with acquisition times between 6 and 15 s are used while respiration is interrupted [37]. The T1-weighted MR sequences, as are used clinically, provide a qualitative visualization of the temperature distribution within the target region. Although temperature resolution is not in the range of 1°C, the region with temperatures above 60°C can clearly be identified so that the actual margin of irreversible tissue damage can be predicted. This has been demonstrated by comparison with fiber optic temperature measurements and a histological examination of in vitro samples [37]. Nevertheless, it is evident that maintaining a significant safety margin around a malignant tumor should always be aimed for. Using MRI for on-line therapy control of LITT provides information about the following parameters, therefore enabling a treatment which is safe: (1) position of the active applicator tips; (2) geometric configuration of sensible structures and large vessels with respect to the applicators; (3) dynamics of heat dissipation, and (4) complete destruction of the target.

It should also be mentioned that there have been a few investigations on applying CT as an on-line control for LITT (F. Wacker, personal commun.).

However, the results showed that a prediction of the actual thermal lesion size is not possible because the absorption properties of the X-ray radiation do not show a significant thermal dependency. Only regions far above 100°C with significant vaporization showed a signal change due to the reduced density. Consequently, CT cannot be recommended as on-line monitoring for LITT.

Besides on-line control, the post-interventional evaluation of the treatment success, i.e. complete thermal destruction of the target tissue, is also an important task. Here, MRI can also be seen as the gold standard. In most LITT protocols a contrast-enhanced MRI study 24–48 h after therapy is established because residual tumor tissue can easily be distinguished from the thermal lesion and the surrounding healthy tissue [38, 39]. However, images acquired later than 48 h after therapy are more difficult to interpret because the natural tissue reaction may interfere with the residual tumor.

Conclusion and Future Aspects of Laser-Induced Thermotherapy

It has be shown that the technical prerequisites for LITT are on a high and evaluated level. This includes laser systems and laser applicators, puncture systems, monitoring systems and therapy planning. Consequently, routine and wide use of LITT for selected indications will be the next step. The expansion of the clinical indications for LITT will be one of the major goals for the near future.

Development tasks on the technical side are related to a further improvements in the instrumentation used for LITT. As mentioned, new technology employing thermo-sensitive sonography as a monitoring tool shows promising preliminary results. On the other hand, optimized sequences for MRI are still under development, providing high resolution thermal on-line mapping with a level of precision better than 3°C, graphically false color representation, and automated moving artifact compensation. Another promising technology is the introduction of virtual methods in surgery and radiology. The measurement of high resolution datasets using MRI or CT and the application of sophisticated algorithms provide the rendering of important structures such as tumors, vessels, bones, and others. A three-dimensional representation of the target region will help the physician to plan therapy and find optimized puncture tracks with minimal side effects. Also the combination of three-dimensional data sets with models of interstitial radiation planning is under current investigation so that the entire therapy will become predictable on the basis of real patient data.

A combination of the previous techniques with fast puncture monitoring and optically tracked puncture instruments will support the physician when approaching the target region. A planned path can be displayed on an overhead screen and each deviation of the instrument will be indicated. This technique is already available in neurosurgery and appears to be a promising tool for other regions such as the liver.

However, laser light is not the only energy source available for in situ ablation. In addition to cryosurgery, the application of monopolar and bipolar radio frequency current is also under investigation for various clinical indications. Therefore, it will be fascinating to see how in situ ablation techniques will gain significant importance in surgical and radiological departments.

References

1   Bown SG: Phototherapy of tumours. World J Surg 1983;7:700–709.
2   Germer CT, Albrecht D, Roggan A, Isbert C, Buhr HJ: Experimental study of laparascopic laser-induced thermotherapy for liver tumors. Br J Surg 1997;84:317–320.
3   Breasted JH: The Edwin Smith Surgical Papyrus. Chicago, University of Chicago, 1930, vol 1.
4   Henriques FCJ, Moritz AR: Studies of thermal injuries. I: The conduction of heat to and through the skin and the temperature attained therein. Am J Pathol 1947;23:531–549.
5   Holm A, Bradley E, Aldrete JS: Hepatic resection of metastases from colorectal carcinoma. Morbidity, mortality and pattern of recurrence. Ann Surg 1989;209:428–434.
6   Sherman DM, Weichselbaum R, Order SE, Cloud L, Trey C, Piro AJ: Palliation of hepatic metastases. Cancer 1978;41:2013–2017.
7   Kemeny N: Review of regional therapy of liver metastases in colorectal cancer. Semin Oncol 1992;19:155–162.
8   Rougier P, Laplanche A, Huguier M, Hay JM, Ollivier JM, Escat J, Salmon R, Julien M, Roullet M, Audy JC, Gallot D: Hepatic arterial infusion of floxuridine in patients with liver metastases from colorectal carcinoma: Long-term results of a prospective randomized trial. J Clin Oncol 1992; 10:1112–1118.
9   Steele G Jr, Bleday R, Mayer RJ, Lindblad A, Petrelli N, Weaver D: A prospective evaluation of hepatic resection for colorectal carcinoma metastases to the liver: Gastrointestinal Tumor Study Group Protocol 6584. J Clin Oncol 1991;9:1105–1112.
10 Vogl TJ, Straub R, Eichler K, Mack MG: Malignant liver tumors treated with MR imaging-guided laser-induced thermotherapy: experience with complications in 899 patients. Radiology 2002; 225:367–377.
11 Bowman HF, Cravalho EG, Woods M: Theory, measurement and application of thermal properties of biological tissue. Annu Rev Biophys Bioeng 1975;4:43–80.
12 Albrecht D, Germer CT, Isbert C, Ritz JP, Roggan A, Müller G, Buhr HJ: Interstitial laser coagulation: Evaluation of the effect of normal liver blood perfusion and the application mode on lesion size. Lasers Surg Med 1998;23:40–47.
13 Parrish JA: New concepts in therapeutic photomedicine: Photochemistry, optical targeting and the therapeutic window. J Invest Dermatol 1981;77:45–50.
14 Roggan A: Dosimetrie thermischer Laseranwendungen in der Medizin – Untersuchung der optischen Gewebeeigenschaften und physikalisch-mathematische Modellentwicklung; in Müller G, Berlien HP (eds): Fortschritte in der Lasermedizin. Landsberg, Ecomed, 1997, vol 16, pp 96–115.
15 Costello AJ, Agarwal DK, Crowe HR, Lynch WJ: Evaluation of interstitial diode laser therapy for treatment of benign prostatic hyperplasia. Tech Urol 1999;5:202–206.
16 Berlien HP, Müller G (eds): Angewandte Lasermedizin, Handbuch für Praxis und Klinik. Landsberg, Ecomed, 1989.
17 Stevenson HN: The effect of heat upon tumor tissue. J Cancer Res 1990;4:54–60.

18   Welch AJ: The thermal response of laser irradiated tissue. IEEE J Quantum Electronics 1984; 2012:1471–1481.

19   Philipp C, Rhode E, Berlien HP: Treatment of congenital vascular disorders (CVD) with laser-induced interstitial thermotherapy (LITT); in Müller G, Roggan A (eds): Laser-Induced Interstitial Thermotherapy. Bellingham, SPIE Press, 1995, pp 443–458.

20   Frank F, Hessel S: Technische Voraussetzungen für die interstitielle Thermotherapie mit dem Nd: YAG-Laser. Lasermedizin 1990;10:36–40.

21   Muschter R, Hofstetter A: Technique and results of interstitial laser coagulation. World J Urol 1995;13:109–114.

22   Roggan A, Albrecht D, Berlien HP, Beuthan J, Fuchs B, Germer C, Mesecke v. Rheinbaben I, Rygiel R, Schründer S, Müller G: Application equipment for intraoperative and percutaneous laser-induced interstitial thermotherapy; in Müller G, Roggan A (eds): Laser-Induced Interstitial Thermotherapy. Bellingham, SPIE Press, 1995, pp 224–248.

23   Germer CT, Albrecht D, Isbert C, Ritz J, Roggan A, Buhr HJ: Diffusing fibre tip for minimally invasive treatment of liver tumours by interstitial laser coagulation (ILC): An experimental ex vivo study. Lasers Med Sci 1999;14:32–39.

24   Vogl TJ, Muller PK, Mack MG, Straub R, Engelmann K, Neuhaus P: Liver metastases: Interventional therapeutic techniques and results, state of the art. Eur Radiol 1999;9:675–684.

25   Wacker FK, Cholewa D, Roggan A, Schilling A, Waldschmidt J, Wolf KJ: Vascular lesions in children: Percutaneous MR imaging-guided interstitial Nd:YAG laser therapy – Preliminary experience. Radiology 1998:208:789–794.

26   Vogl TJ, Mack MG, Roggan A, Straub R, Eichler KC, Müller PK, Knappe V, Felix R: Internally cooled power laser for MR-guided interstitial laser-induced thermotherapy of liver lesions: Initial clinical results. Radiology 1998;209:381–385.

27   Germer CT, Isbert C, Albrecht D, Roggan A, Pelz J, Ritz JP, Müller G, Buhr HJ: Laser-induced thermotherapy combined with hepatic arterial embolization in the treatment of liver tumors in a rat tumor model. Ann Surg 1999;320:55–62.

28   Wacker F, Reither K, Ritz JP, Roggan A, Germer CT, Wolf KJ: MR-guided interstitial laser-induced thermotherapy of hepatic metastases combined with arterial blood flow reduction: Technique and first clinical results in an open MR system. J Mag Res Imaging 2001;13:31–36.

29   Rau B, Wust P, Tilly W, Gellermann J, Harder C, Riess H, Budach V, Felix R, Schlag PM: Preoperative radiochemotherapy in locally advanced or recurrent rectal cancer: Regional radiofrequency hyperthermia correlates with clinical parameters. Int J Radiat Oncol Biol Phys 2000; 48:381–391.

30   Roggan A, Knappe V, Ritz JP, Germer CT, Isbert C, Wacker F, Müller G: 3D-Bestrahlungsplanung für die laserinduzierte Thermotherapie (LITT). Z Med Phys 2000;10:157–167.

31   Roggan A, Müller G: Dosimetry and computer based irradiation planning for laser-induced interstitial thermotherapy (LITT); in Müller G, Roggan A (eds): Laser-Induced Interstitial Thermotherapy. Bellingham, SPIE Press, 1995, pp 114–157.

32   Dachman AH, McGehee JA, Beam TE: US-guided percutaneous laser ablation of liver tissue in a chronic pig model. Radiology 1990;176:128–133.

33   Bosman S, Phoa SSK, Bosma A, van Gemert MJC: Effect of percutaneous interstitial thermal laser on normal liver of pigs: Sonographic and histopathological correlations. Br J Surg 1991;78:572–575.

34   Mesecke-von Rheinbaben I: Monitoringverfahren zur Überwachung koagulativer Gewebeeffekte der interstitiellen Thermotherapie – Untersuchungen zur Eignung der Doppler-Sonographie und optischer Durchleuchtungsverfahren; in Müller G, Berlien HP (eds): Fortschritte in der Lasermedizin. Landsberg, Ecomed, 2001, vol 23, pp 178–186.

35   Jolesz FA, Bleier AR, Jakab P, Ruenzel PW, Huttl K, Jako GJ: MR imaging of laser tissue interaction. Radiology 1988;168:853–857.

36   Gewiese B, Beuthan J, Fobbe F, Stiller D, Müller G, Boese-Landgraf J, Wolf KJ, Deimling M: Magnetic resonance imaging-controlled laser-induced interstitial thermotherapy. Invest Radiol 1994;29:345–351.

37   Vogl TJ, Weinhold N, Mack MG, Müller PK, Scholz WR, Straub R, Roggan A, Felix R: Verification of MR thermometry by means of an in vivo intralesional, fluorooptic temperature measurement for laser-induced thermotherapy of liver metastases. Fortschr Röntgenstr 1998;169:182–188.

38 Isbert C, Germer CT, Albrecht D, Schilling A, Heiniche A, Ritz J-P, Roggan A, Buhr HJ: Kontrastmittelgestützte MRT als Monitoring Verfahren des Follow-up nach laserinduzierter Thermotherapie – Eine experimentelle Korrelationsanalyse in vivo. Endoskopie heute 1997;10: 145–146.

39 Germer CT, Isbert CM, Albrecht D, Ritz JP, Schilling A, Roggan A, Wolf KJ, Müller G, Buhr HJ: Laser-induced thermotherapy for the treatment of liver metastasis. Surg Endosc 1998;12:1317–1325.

Dr. med Jörg-Peter Ritz
Chirurgische Klinik und Poliklinik I, Allgemein-, Gefäss- und Thoraxchirurgie
Charité – Universitätsmedizin Berlin, Campus Benjamin Franklin
Freie- und Humboldt-Universität zu Berlin,
Hindenburgdamm 30, DE–12200 Berlin (Germany)
Tel. +49 30 8445 2543, Fax +49 30 8445 2740, E-Mail ritz@medizin.fu-berlin.de

Author Index

Subject Index

Rectal cancer
  digital rectal examination, staging 29
  endoluminal ultrasound 30, 38
  liver metastases, *see* Colorectal liver
    metastases
  magnetic resonance imaging
    advantages 1, 10
    circumferential resection margin
      prediction 5, 6, 30, 31
    coils/resolution 2, 3
    radiation therapy patient precautions
      7, 9, 10
    recurrent cancer 38, 39
    staging accuracy 2, 3, 7, 30, 31
  postoperative radiochemotherapy 41,
    52–55
  preoperative radiation therapy
    advantages/limitations 13, 14, 21
    approaches 14
    curable tumors 24, 26
    delayed-surgery outcomes 25
    dose escalation/tumor response 26
    local control, surgery 25
    short-course therapy outcomes 18–21,
      33, 34
    sphincter preservation outcomes 25, 26
  preoperative radiochemotherapy
    advantages/limitations 13, 14, 21
    resectable tumors 17, 18
    sphincter preservation, low-lying
      tumors 16, 17
    T4 rectal cancer 14, 15
  recurrent cancer
    computed tomography criteria 38
    external beam radiotherapy,
      with/without chemotherapy 58
    fractionation schedules, radiotherapy
      62–64
    high linear energy transfer
      radiotherapy 62
    hyperthermia, radiochemotherapy
      61, 62
    imaging 37–39
    intensity-modulated radiotherapy
      58, 59

    intra-arterial chemotherapy/
      radiotherapy 62
    intraoperative high-dose-rate
      brachytherapy 61
    intraoperative radiotherapy 52–55,
      59–61
    multicenter analysis
      abdominoperineal resection versus
        low anterior resection 44, 47, 48
      clinical features 44, 48
      infiltration sites 42–44
      initial staging 42, 43
      sites of recurrence 44–47
      study design 42
      study limitations 48, 49
    radiosensitizers 64
    resectability 37
  total mesorectal excision surgery
    circumferential resection margin 28, 29
    preoperative radiation therapy 24, 26,
      33, 34
    quality factors 32
    staging 29–31
    technique 31, 32

Stereotactic radiation therapy, liver
  metastases
  accuracy/safety margin 101
  body frame 100
  morbidity 102
  outcomes 102, 103
  prospects 103, 104
  study design 101, 102

Total mesorectal excision surgery (TME)
  circumferential resection margin
    28, 29
  preoperative radiation therapy 24, 26,
    33, 34
  quality factors 32
  staging, rectal cancer 29–31
  technique 31, 32

Ultrasound, endoluminal, rectal cancer
  30, 38